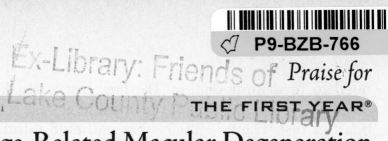

Praise for

THE FIRST YEAR®

Age-Related Macular Degeneration

"Daniel Roberts does not just give AMD patients and those who care for them all the facts and resources they need, in a highly readable and often entertaining form. By his own example he also shows them that, no matter how bitter the lemons of the diagnosis, they too can make lemonade by becoming patient experts themselves."

—GISLIN DAGNELIE, PHD,
Lions Vision Research & Rehabilitation Center,
Johns Hopkins University School of Medicine

"At last a book on macular degeneration for the general public that treats the reader as an intelligent individual capable of understanding the concepts and information presented. Daniel Roberts does a wonderful job of explaining macular degeneration, its affects on vision function and what can be done to lessen its impact on one's life."

—JOSEPH H. MAINO, O.D.,
Fellow of the Academy of American
Ophthalmology, Kansas City VA Medical Center

"A comprehensive work that I would recommend to anyone who has AMD, to their family and others, and to all eye care practitioners as a resource both for themselves and for their patients who are just developing the condition."

—ROY COLE, O.D., Director,
The Jewish Guild for the Blind

"If you've been told you have macular degeneration, and that nothing can be done about it, here is a book you need to read immediately. *The First Year*®—*Age-Related Macular Degeneration* will set your mind at ease and your heart at rest. Daniel Roberts has gathered information and wisdom that will show you everything that can be done. Learn the basic facts, read the stories of others, try out the useful tips and follow up on all the resources available to you. It will absolutely change the way you look at this disease."

—JUDITH DELGADO, Director,
The Macular Degeneration Partnership

"Rather than concentrating all the clinical material in one large section, Daniel Roberts presents smaller, more approachable units on clinical aspects of macular degeneration as well as low vision approaches and patient experience. At the same time, he presents a thorough discussion of each topic, so that the reader gets an up to date and accurate picture of macular degeneration in digestible bites. I'm sure it will help many, many patients and families affected by macular degeneration."

—JANET S. SUNNESS, M.D.,
Retina and Low Vision Specialist Medical Director,
Richard E. Hoover Rehabilitation Services for Low Vision and Blindness, Greater Baltimore Medical Center

"A reassuring and sensible in-depth conversation with a knowledgeable friend at the time it is most needed."

—MARY JAY CLOUGH, LCSW, ACSW,
The Jewish Guild for the Blind

"An indispensable guide for those with macular degeneration. Clear and to the point, this is a book I will recommend to others for all of its valuable information."

—JOHN BLAKEFIELD,
living with age-related macular degeneration

DANIEL L. ROBERTS is the founding director of MD Support, Inc. and the National Low Vision Support Group. These non-profit organizations offer support and information to people around the world who are affected by macular degeneration. Roberts provides free presentations about vision impairment for schools, community organizations, and support groups, and he leads workshops at the University of Missouri at Kansas City, Longview Community College, and the Mid-Continent Public Libraries. Roberts is the recipient of the 2004 Distinguished Service Award presented by the American Optometric Association Low Vision Rehabilitation Section. He lives with his wife in Grandview, Missouri.

The Complete FIRST YEAR® Series

THE FIRST YEAR®

Age-Related Macular Degeneration

An Essential Guide for the Newly Diagnosed

Daniel L. Roberts

Foreword by Lylas G. Mogk, MD

Da Capo
∞
LIFE
LONG

A MEMBER OF THE PERSEUS BOOKS GROUP

Designed by Pauline Neuwirth, Neuwirth and Associates, Inc.
Set in 14 point Fairfield LH by the Perseus Books Group

Cataloging-in-Publication data for this book is available from the Library of Congress.

ISBN: 978-1-56924-286-5

Published by Da Capo Press
A Member of the Perseus Books Group
www.dacapopress.com

Da Capo Press books are available at special discounts for bulk purchases in the U.S. by corporations, institutions, and other organizations. For more information, please contact the Special Markets Department at the Perseus Books Group, 2300 Chestnut Street, Suite 200, Philadelphia, PA, 19103, or call (800) 810-4145, extension 5000, or e-mail special.markets@perseusbooks.com.

10 9 8 7 6 5 4

To the original dozen members of the
MDList who helped and encouraged me
during my "First Year." Most of all
to my wife, Christina, who continues to
offer her strength when I misplace mine.

In Memoriam

Donna Broadstock (1935–2003)
James Dillon, OD (1944–2002)
Irving Faust (1928–2004)

Contents

CONTENTS

Foreword

by Lylas G. Mogk, MD

IT IS a shock to discover that the problem with reading the newspaper is not in your glasses, but in your eyes. The diagnosis of macular degeneration and the loss of any amount of central vision is a stunning experience for sighted adults. We are used to conveying and absorbing vast amounts of information visually or in print. Our buildings, offices, homes, and appliances are designed with the assumption that everyone has full vision, and our love affair with automobiles has produced urban geographies in most parts of the country that require everyone to drive. Those of us who are sighted routinely assume full sight in others and practice many social behaviors that are sight-based, such as giving directions by pointing, and responding to comments with facial expressions. If we had tried to build a society and a culture that would condition us to be totally dependent on our vision in every respect—physically, functionally, socially, and emotionally—we really could not have done a better job. As a result, sighted adults are strikingly ill adapted to vision loss.

This situation is compounded for the central vision loss of macular degeneration, because central vision occupies a dominant position in our consciousness. Central vision is what we see when we look directly at something—the words we are reading, or our child's face, for example. The macula, which is responsible for central vision, is a very small spot at the center of our retina, but its visual message occupies half the area of our brain that is devoted to interpreting vision. Peripheral vision is everything we see that we are not looking directly at. It is important vision that allows us to walk in a crowded area without bumping into others, but it does not help us read the newspaper. We can lose a lot of peripheral vision without noticing, but we are immediately aware of a little bit of central vision loss.

It is an irony that central vision loss, as striking as it is to the individual, is completely invisible to others. If you have central vision loss from macular degeneration, you look fine, like you always did. You make eye contact and walk around well. You see a lot, so others, including physicians, may underestimate the impact of your change in vision. Family and friends may conclude that you are just seeing what you want to see. ("Grandpa," my daughter used to say to my father, who had advanced age-related macular degeneration [AMD], "I think you're fooling me. How come you could see a little button on the floor but you can't tell who I am?") Or they may over-estimate, and become fearful and overprotective.

The combination of central vision loss and the sparing of peripheral vision (the ability to see everything around the edges of your vision that you are not looking at directly) makes it difficult to explain why you can see some things but not others. Our vocabulary of vision contributes to this by offering the limited choice of "sight" or "blindness," with the implication that blindness means no vision at all. People with macular degeneration do not fit into this dichotomy: on the one hand, with a little contrast loss from early macular degeneration you may be very aware that your vision is affected and that some important details are obscured; on the other hand, with even advanced AMD you retain full peripheral vision, you are not blind, and never will be. The intermediate term "hard of seeing" coined by Lorraine Marchi, LHD, affords a more accurate perception of central vision loss from macular degeneration as a real challenge to our daily lives but one we can meet.

To meet this challenge and continue living fully with central vision loss, we need to be empowered with knowledge about macular degeneration and patterns of vision loss, creative strategies for coping emotionally, techniques and tools for using remaining vision efficiently, information about the spectrum of resources, and support from those who share the experience.

This book reaches out to you to offer all of these. It is a testament to the impact of early vision loss, but also to the fact that you can live fully and vibrantly in spite of vision loss at any level. It provides a wealth of empowering knowledge, important information, perceptive observations, compelling stories, and practical suggestions

from patients and professionals alike. It is spiced
throughout with enormous empathy, kindly tough love,
inspiring enthusiasm, and the endearing humor of Dan
Roberts and the people who inhabit his worldwide AMD
community—all of whom are walking this path with you.

LYLAS G. MOGK, MD, is an ophthalmologist; medical director of the
Henry Ford Health System Visual Rehabilitation and Research
Center in Grosse Pointe and Livonia, Michigan; coauthor of *Macular Degeneration: The Complete Guide to Saving and Maximizing Your Sight*; and chair of the American Academy of Ophthalmology
Vision Rehabilitation Committee.

Introduction

IN 1993 I was in my twenty-second year of public school music teaching—fully intending to reach full retirement by my mid-fifties. Then, in 1994, my entire future took a detour. The visual spots that I first thought were caused by temporary "burn-in" from the bright light of the copy machine turned out to be much more. When the spots didn't go away and I started noticing cars on the highway disappearing into them, I decided it was time to see a doctor. The next bright flashes were into my dilated eyes as the examiner took photographs of my retinas. The diagnosis that followed was the most difficult news I have ever received. My central vision was deteriorating. To help slow down progression of the disease, the doctor injected a steroid into the tissue around my worst eye and told me there was nothing more that could be done. I asked him if my vision might last until retirement. He gave me my answer by smiling sympathetically and crossing his fingers as if to say "good luck." Then he left the room, making that the last time I saw him, because I chose to look elsewhere for the answer to my problem.

The Internet was still new, but I thought perhaps I could find help through that strange invention called the World Wide Web. After weeks of searching through the tangle of disorganized information and dead ends (I was sure that's why it's called a "web"), I discovered a little group of about a dozen people who had found one another and formed an e-mail support group called MDList. They had all lost central vision from macular degeneration, and they took me under their wings.

Cut to the present. My left eye has progressed to total central vision loss, and my right eye is holding at 20/40 corrected. I had expected it to be worse by this time, which is why I opted for early retirement to run my own performing arts school on my own schedule. What I didn't expect was the direction my life took.

I am now the owner of MDList, which has grown to nearly four hundred people from more than twenty countries. Over the past twelve years we have gathered more than 650 Internet pages of documents, and our Web site averages over 3 million hits annually from patients, family members, and eye care specialists who are looking for information and support.

In order to better reach out to the millions of people who are in need of help, we incorporated in 1998 as a nonprofit charity under the name Macular Degeneration Support and acquired a twelve-member professional advisory board to guide us. Within five years of diagnosis with a disease that I thought would destroy my future, I found myself following a new and unimaginably rewarding career as director of one of the leading low vision organizations in the world.

Our primary goal is to ensure that no one will ever be alone with this disease. No newly diagnosed patient should ever walk out of a doctor's office with nowhere to go and no one to turn to. Everyone should have immediate answers to the "Big Ten" questions:

What is AMD, and how did I get it?
What should I expect?
What can I do to improve my visual health?
How can I live successfully with visual impairment?
What types of doctors should I be seeing?
What kinds of surgeries or interventions are available?
What treatments or potential cures are there?
What are my rights as a visually impaired person?
Should I join a clinical trial?
Where can I find more help?

The First Year—Age-Related Macular Degeneration is a compilation of the knowledge and experiences of patients, doctors, social workers, nutritionists, and low vision rehabilitation specialists who deal with macular degeneration on a daily basis. Everything is here to provide you, your family, and your friends with an understanding of your condition and your needs. Many people from our AMD community, both laypeople and professionals, have contributed personal stories and informational articles to these pages to empower you with the weapons you need for waging an all-out war against the emotional onslaught of potential vision loss.

Based upon the course of most patients' needs, the book guides you through the answers you want, and in the order you want them. You will be taken through your first week day by day to respond to your most *immediate* concerns. Each of the days will walk you through easy-to-understand topics (Learning) followed by ways you can put the information into practice (Living).

After the first seven days, the chapters are organized by weeks and then by months, as the focus broadens into issues that are secondary to your initial needs. Learning and Living, by that time, will be presented simultaneously, because you will have developed a solid foundation of knowledge. Learning will therefore require less of your time, which can then be spent on maintaining and improving your quality of life.

An equally important part of the book is the resource section at the back. In addition to a list of AMD organizations in the final chapter, the appendixes provide additional contact information about state agencies, financial assistance organizations, dealers in low vision devices, books in large print and audio, and drugs to avoid. You will also find a complete glossary of ophthalmic terms, with definitions you can understand.

In other words, *The First Year—Age-Related Macular Degeneration* is intended to be a complete resource that will help you deal with every aspect of age-related macular degeneration and related diseases that may lead to central vision loss. It is more than a book about AMD. It is a reference to which you will want to return often as your needs evolve. You will also want to pass it along to other people in your life. By helping to educate your immediate family and social circle, you will build around yourself a strong fortress of knowledge and support. That will be of immense comfort to both you and them.

On behalf of everyone you will meet in these chapters, thank you for joining our worldwide community of caring and information. Hopefully, the sum of our parts will keep you whole. Your life is changing, and we hope it will be for the better by our contribution to it.

DANIEL L. ROBERTS

What Is AMD, and How Did You Get It?

FOCAL POINTS:

- *Your worst enemy is fear of the unknown.*
- *Knowledge is power.*

YOU HAVE been diagnosed with **age-related macular degeneration (AMD)**. This means that you may lose part of your vision. Since you depend upon your eyesight for nearly everything you do, the thought of losing it can upset you as much as the thought of losing a member of your family. That is a normal reaction, but you don't have to let it consume you.

This book is designed to help you understand and deal with AMD. By learning about every facet of the disease, much of your fear will be eased. By learning how to deal with it, you can maximize your remaining vision and retain much of your independence.

You can manage this unexpected detour. AMD is not life threatening, nor is it painful. Millions of people share it with you, and scientists are working hard to cure it. You can draw strength from that kind of support. Trust what you have already learned in your life: that nothing is as bad as you expect, especially when you have lots of people to guide you and share it with you.

You are not alone.

Many of those people are within these pages, so fix yourself a cup of hot chocolate or a glass of red wine (both drinks are good for your eyes), and find a comfortable chair. The first day is the hardest, but you'll soon see how much easier the journey can become.

The bad news and the good news

First, the bad news. As you have probably been told, AMD can destroy central vision in both eyes, making it difficult or impossible to read, sign checks, recognize faces, and pass driver's license examinations.

The good news is that AMD progresses very slowly in most cases, affecting *only your central vision*. No matter how far the disease advances, your **peripheral (side) vision** will remain intact.

You will not go blind from AMD.

The facts about AMD

Age-related macular degeneration (AMD) is a progressive disease of the **retina** wherein the light-sensing **cells** in the central area of vision stop working and eventually die. The disease is thought to be caused by a combination of genetics and environment, and it is most common in people who are age sixty and over. AMD is the leading cause of **visual impairment** in adults. Most sources estimate that as many as 8.5 million people in the United States have it, and as many as 200,000 new cases are diagnosed annually.[1]

Other less common types of macular degeneration, which are hereditary and can affect younger people, are Best's disease, Stargardt's disease, and Sorsby's disease. Collectively, these types are called **juvenile macular degeneration**. If you are under fifty-five years old, but your macular degeneration is not in one of these forms, your condition might be called **early onset AMD.** Other diseases of the retina and extreme **myopia** (nearsightedness) can also result in degeneration of the macula. These conditions are not to be confused with AMD, but the end result, loss of central vision, can be the same. This book will still prove helpful to you if you have myopic MD or one of the many other forms.

Even with advanced AMD, you can do well with little or no assistance by using *low vision devices, electronic magnification,* and *computer software.* This kind of technology will allow you to continue leading an independent and productive life.

AMD is classified into two types: **dry** (also called **atrophic)** and **wet** (also called **exudative** or

neovascular). You will want to understand the difference so you can identify proper treatment strategies.

Dry (atrophic) AMD

Most cases of AMD are the dry form, distinguished by yellowish deposits of lipids (cellular waste), called **drusen**, in your retina. The material that makes up drusen is usually carried away by the same blood vessels that bring nutrients to your retina. This process, however, is diminished in AMD.

Some of the suspected reasons for drusen are *inflammation, inadequate blood circulation* in the retina, and *premature aging of the photoreceptor cells,* due to genetic deficiencies. In addition, science has shown that *environmental, behavioral*, and *dietary factors* can contribute to the progress of the disease. You will learn about these in Day 4.

Dry AMD may occur in three stages in one or both eyes:

Early Dry AMD is identified by several small cellular waste deposits (drusen) in your medium-sized drusen, with no obvious symptoms or vision loss.

Intermediate Dry AMD is identified by many medium-sized drusen or one or more large, irregular-shaped drusen (called **soft drusen**). Symptoms may include a blurred or **blind spot** (**scotoma**) or distortion of images in your central field of vision, as seen in Figure 1. Also, you may need more light and higher contrast for seeing.

Advanced Dry AMD involves drusen as described above, plus a breakdown of light-sensing *photo-*

receptor cells and surrounding tissue in the macula. Scotomas may become larger and distortion more severe, eventually encompassing the entire central field. This would make detail vision impossible, forcing you to rely upon your peripheral field for sight.

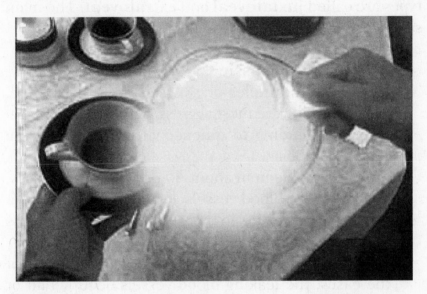

Figure 1. How a person sees with advanced AMD

At the time of this writing, no cure or **FDA-approved** treatments are available for dry macular degeneration. Scientists are, however, studying the value of several experimental therapies. You will learn about these in Weeks 2 and 3.

Wet (exudative or neovascular) AMD

In about 10 to 15 percent of AMD cases, newly formed, immature blood vessels grow from the **choroid** layer of the retina and leak into the spaces above and below the photoreceptor cone cells. This process, called **choroidal neovascularization (CNV)**, can damage the cones and cause permanent central vision loss.

Nearly 90 percent of wet MD cases are of the **subfoveal** type. This means the offending vessels are beneath the **fovea**, or very center of the macula. Other types are called **juxtafoveal** and **extrafoveal**. The main subtypes of subfoveal wet AMD are:

> **Predominantly classic CNV.** Seen in about 25 percent of cases, the leaking vessels are well defined. This is usually the most aggressive form of subfoveal wet MD, leading to quicker vision loss than the other subtypes.
>
> **Occult CNV.** Seen in about 40 percent of the cases, the offending blood vessels are not readily defined. Occult AMD results in the slowest rate of vision loss of the three subtypes.
>
> **Minimally classic CNV.** Seen in about 35 percent of the cases, the leaking blood vessels occupy half or less of the area of the entire lesion. It has a slower rate of vision loss than predominantly classic, but is faster than occult.

Neovascularization is becoming better understood as research progresses. The basic problem is that bleeding damages retinal tissues and causes scarring that can block vision. Neovascularization can be a reparative response in other parts of the body. It is ironic that in the macula, it causes destructive scarring leading to central vision loss.

How your diagnosis was made

A decision about your treatment was probably made using either **fluorescein angiography (FA)** or **ocular coherence tomography (OCT)**, and perhaps both.

For FA, *fluorescein dye* is injected into a vein in the patient's hand. The dye travels to the retina, where it causes the blood to glow, allowing photographs to be taken to determine the location of any leakage that may be present. The camera's bright flashes can be uncomfortable, but the procedure is not harmful, and it doesn't take long. The patient must sign a form prior to FA, signifying that **informed consent** has been given.

Diagnosis using OCT requires no dye injection or flashing lights. This newer method uses an optical device to generate a cross-section image of the retinal layers, allowing for measurement of tissue thickness. Swelling of the retinal tissue is one indication of AMD.

Your doctor also performed direct examination of your **dilated** eyes using a **slit lamp** (a kind of lighted microscope). An experienced eye care specialist can identify many of the symptoms of AMD using this method alone.

Another diagnostic tool that is not yet in wide use is **scanning laser ophthalmoscopy (SLO).** This involves a narrow low-intensity laser beam that quickly scans the surface of the retina, creating images on a computer monitor. This is an improvement over FA, in that it does not flash a bright light into the patient's eye.

What to expect

The foremost question in your mind right now is probably, "How much time do I have before I lose my central vision?"

That's a good question. Unfortunately, there is no good answer. Each person's genetic makeup, diet, behavior, and environment are different. Some people move into the advanced stages of AMD within months. Others slowly progress over years and may never reach the end stage. That's why the best advice is to learn as much as you can about the disease, follow your doctor's advice, and keep a positive attitude.

> **Prepare for the worst, but expect the best.**

By reading this book, you are preparing to meet the enemy armed with every weapon available. You will also learn that, at its worst, AMD by itself will not leave you sightless. So as you hold on to that promise, here are some straightforward facts for you:

If you have the dry form of AMD,

Then . . .

your central vision will deteriorate *slowly.* You will have time to adapt, both physically and emotionally. You will *not* wake up one morning as a blind person.

If you develop the wet form of AMD,

Then . . .

your central vision could go quickly. Get to the doctor within four or five days, however, and your chances are good that your sight can be saved. Again, you will learn about these treatments later in Weeks 2 and 3.

If you reach end-stage AMD,

Then . . .

you will not be able to read without high magnification, nor will you be able to distinguish most colors, recognize faces at a distance, or safely drive a vehicle. You *will*, however, be able to move about without mobility aids or a guide animal and will get around so well that you will not have to explain to strangers that you are visually impaired, unless you find it useful (see pp.12–13).

If you live alone and wish to continue doing so,

Then . . .

rehabilitation specialists are prepared to help you adapt your environment for living successfully with low vision. More about that in Day 5.

Focus on the Facts

You've been given a great deal of information on this first day. To help you put it all together, here are the main points:

Age-related macular degeneration (AMD) is a progressive disease of the retina wherein the light-sensing cells in the central area of vision stop working and eventually die.

AMD progresses very slowly in most cases and affects only your central vision.

Even with advanced AMD, you can do well with little or no assistance by using low vision devices, electronic magnification, and computer software. Low vision rehabilitation training is highly recommended.

AMD is classified into two types: dry (also called atrophic) and wet (also called exudative or neovascular).

Your doctor probably sees drusen in your retina, which could be of the hard or the soft type.

Dry AMD may occur in three stages in one or both eyes: early, intermediate, and advanced.

The main subtypes of subfoveal wet AMD are predominantly classic, occult, and minimally classic.

In addition to direct observation with a magnifier, your diagnosis was made using fluorescein angiography (FA), ocular coherence tomography (OCT), scanning laser ophthalmoscopy (SLO), or maybe all three.

living

Help Others Understand

NOW YOU are acquainted with this thing that is happening to you. But what about your family and friends? How and what do you tell them? Why don't they want to talk about it, and why don't they understand how it makes you feel? What do you say to people when they ask what they can do to help? What do you say to your granddaughter when she asks why you never drive her anywhere? How do you handle that woman in the grocery store who says loudly enough for everyone to hear, "Hey, if you can't count change faster than that, get a credit card"? This section and the people it introduces will help you around some of those awkward times.

Susan's story

I was pacing slowly down the sidewalk so that I wouldn't trip over that crack like I did the day before. My mail was in one hand, and I shaded my eyes with the other. My sunglasses were the recommended kind, but I realized I should have worn my big hat to keep the sun from glaring off them.

I heard the *clack-clack* of skateboard wheels coming at me head-on. A few years ago, I would have stepped aside, but now I didn't know which way to step. So I just froze in place, hoping the pilot of that conveyance would have good maneuvering skills.

He didn't. He collided with my left hip, and his ride escaped into the street. He ran after it, and I screamed at the sound of a blaring horn and tires scraping on loose gravel.

The boy returned unharmed and slammed his skateboard back onto the concrete walk. He stood in silence for a few seconds—probably scowling at me. Then, with a push of a toe, he was off again, leaving me standing there wondering how I would get my mail from then on.

AMD: *An invisible disease*

The boy in Susan's story was inconsiderate. On the other hand, maybe he thought *she* was the inconsiderate one. Why couldn't she simply have stepped aside as he thought she would, instead of being so stubborn? After all, it was his sidewalk, too. If he had known Susan couldn't see him, would that have changed things? Probably. But what is she supposed to do? Carry a sign? Maybe.

You need to let some people know that you are visually impaired. Maybe you don't have to carry a placard on a stick, but maybe you could carry just the stick. And paint it white. A white cane is the universal symbol of visual impairment. Almost everyone knows what it means, so why not take advantage of that? You may not need a cane to get around, but it can be a very effective way to protect yourself and to explain your sometimes unusual ways. And you have every right to carry one.

You don't have to be blind to carry a cane.

Don't be embarrassed to reveal your visual impairment when necessary. You'll be amazed at how much people will respect your courage and honesty.

Bob's story

I finally agreed to visit a support group at the library, even though I still have pretty good vision and didn't think I needed to be there. Before the meeting, this fellow with a beautiful yellow Labrador struck up a conversation with me. We talked for a while, and then it looked like things were ready to begin. I gave his dog a pat on the head, said, "Excuse me," and headed for a chair.

Then I noticed that my new friend was still talking—to the potted floor plant. He thought I was still there! And that dog was looking at me as if to say, "Get back here, you fool." I got back just in time to hear the fellow say, " . . . but she's on duty, so please avoid petting her." Wow. Two mistakes in less than a minute. I guess I needed to be there after all.

Contrary to the dog's opinion, Bob wasn't a fool. He was just unaware of the basic social courtesies that visually impaired people (**VIP**s) should enjoy. As a VIP himself, it would serve him well to learn them and start putting them into practice.

Here are some rules of etiquette that you might want to pass along. They may not all apply to your situation at this time, but they are good for everyone to know.

Basic Courtesies for the Visually Impaired

Address us by name so that we know you are talking to us.

Speak directly to us, rather than through someone else.

Greet us by giving your name so that we recognize you.

Speak in a natural conversational tone. It is not necessary to speak loudly or to overenunciate.

Feel free to use words that refer to vision. We also use the words "see," "look," "watch," etc. And remember, we are not offended by the term "blind."

Be calm and clear about what to do if you see us encountering a dangerous situation. Saying, "Stop," for example, is better than saying, "Watch out."

If you think we need assistance, ask first. Don't assume that help is needed.

When offering assistance, never take hold of us uninvited. Simply make the offer, and let it be our decision.

Never take hold of a white cane.

Never pet or distract a guide dog while it is on duty.

(Adapted from suggestions by Carl Augusto, president, American Federation for the Blind in New York, and David McGown, executive director, Guild for the Blind in Chicago.)

A script to help you explain

Communicating your situation and how you feel is a good idea, but how do you explain what you see (or don't see)? That's not easy, but it is necessary for the complete understanding of those who care about you.

Some people don't understand, for example, how you can spot a dime on the floor but not see a truck on the highway. They don't know why you don't just get a stronger spectacle prescription if you have trouble reading. It doesn't make sense to them why you need strong light in the house but need to wear sunglasses outdoors. To help you explain, here is a script that works well in most cases:

> "I have macular degeneration, which leads to **visual impairment** (or **low vision**)." ("Visual impairment" and "low vision" are the most acceptable terms for someone with significantly impaired vision that is not correctable with conventional devices.)

> "My vision cannot be improved with regular glasses."

> "Macular degeneration is an incurable disease of the retina that can lead to total central vision loss, but I am not **blind**." (The term "blind" means total lack of light sensitivity by the retina.)

That should be enough to satisfy a passing acquaintance, and you might even want to carry a few copies of it to hand to people who have a need to know. (Like that impatient woman in the grocery store, bless her heart. It will give her something to keep her busy while you count your change.)

Friends and family members may want to know more. If so, here is the next part of your script.

If you experience distortion: "My vision is like looking at a funhouse mirror."

If you have a blind spot: "My vision is like looking through a window that has a spot of petroleum jelly in the middle."

If you experience distortion and have a blind spot: "My vision is like looking at a funhouse mirror that has a spot of petroleum jelly in the middle."

Here is an exercise you can ask others to do that can help you explain the challenges of seeing with advanced AMD. "Close one eye and hold your clenched fist in front of your other eye about nine inches away. Without looking away from your fist, try reading a book or walking about the room."

As you know, words can only go so far. Eventually, you have to show a picture. The photo in Figure 1 is a good example of the end stage of AMD. You might see other representations that show a darker scotoma, but usually images with the blind area are just "not there." The scotoma will often take on the dominant color of the background. This is the brain's attempt at explaining the missing part of your vision. While looking at a ball lying on a green rug, for example, you would see only the green rug.

Knowledge and *support* are key elements in living successfully with AMD. Both elements require effort, but they will pay off in quality of life.

A Message from the AMD Community

Dear Tom,

As an optometrist, I am a huge advocate of people standing up and educating those around them about their vision, but my husband chooses not to do this. Not a soul at work knows he has a vision problem, and he has come up with a million ways to hide it. It frustrates me to no end.

How can anyone understand low vision if no one explains it to them? When people think about vision loss, they picture the blind beggar on the street. How will they ever learn otherwise unless they know someone with a vision impairment who discusses it with them?

How can you ever network with others with vision loss if both you and they are hiding it? You could be crossing paths with others just like you every day and not know it.

Vision loss is an invisible change. No one can tell that anything has happened to you unless you tell them. Just think of the number of misunderstandings that could be avoided.

Dr. Jen

IN A SENTENCE:

> *The best way to fight the emotional trauma of vision loss from AMD is through understanding, an obligation that belongs to both you and the people with whom you interact.*

How Your Eye Is Built

FOCAL POINTS:

▶ *The eyeball is one of nature's most marvelous inventions.*
▶ *AMD is one of many different retinal diseases.*

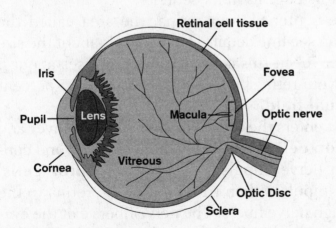

Figure 2. The eyeball

THE FRONT (anterior) part of your **eye** receives and focuses light onto your retina. As seen in Figure 2, the **cornea** is the transparent part of the eyeball, which covers the **iris** and **pupil**. A **tear film** normally coats the cornea, keeping your eye moist. Directly behind the cornea is the **aqueous chamber.** It is filled with a clear fluid for the purpose of maintaining the pressure of the eye.

Your **pupil** is the opening in the center of your eyeball through which light passes. The colored diaphragm surrounding the pupil contracts and expands to adjust for light intensity. This colored part is your **iris**.

The transparent, dual-convex body that focuses light rays onto your retina is the **lens**. It is normally capable of changing shape to allow the eye to focus on both near and distant images.

The **retina**, as seen in Figure 2, is located at the inside back of your eyeball. It captures light like the film in a camera. Film, however, is different, in that it is just as sensitive at its edge as in its center.

Only the center of your retina, the area called the **macula**, can see fine detail. The macula is about the size of the letter "o" in this sentence. It comprises about 5 percent of your retina but accounts for about 35 percent of your **visual field.**

Light first enters the **optic (or nerve) fiber layer** and the **ganglion cell layer**. The light is received and converted into nerve impulses by **photoreceptor cells**. The nerve impulses then travel out of the retina to the brain through nerve fibers. The nerve fibers exit the eyeball at the **optic disc** and reach the brain through the **optic nerve**.

Figure 3 shows the magnified retina as seen by your doctor. The retina, which lines the inside of the eyeball, is essentially transparent, so a doctor can see through all of the layers to the **choroid**. The choroid is where the blood vessels are located, and these vessels give the retina its reddish hue. This also explains why "red eye" often occurs in photographs.

Your examiner, peering through the clear **vitreous fluid** that fills much of your eye, actually looks through the transparent layers of your retina, which lie on top of the **retinal pigment epithelium (RPE)**. The RPE is a single layer of cells that supplies nutrients to the photoreceptors. **Bruch's membrane** separates the RPE from the underlying blood vessels of the choroid. The choroid lies between Bruch's membrane and the eye's tough white outer shell, known as the **sclera.** (See Figure 2.)

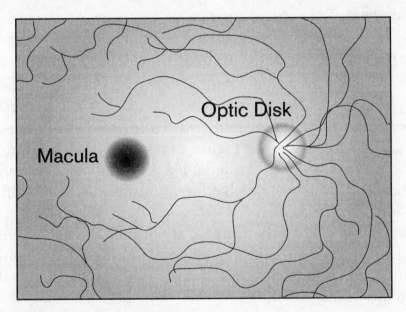

Figure 3. A normal retina

There are two types of photoreceptor cells: the **rod and cone cells**.

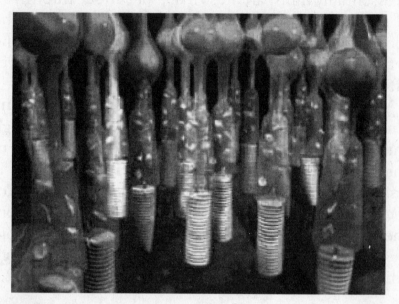

Figure 4. The rod and cone cells

Rods are responsible for **peripheral** and dim light vision. Cones are responsible for central, bright light, fine detail, and **color vision**. The macula has the highest concentration of cone cells, with a few rod cells mixed in. The tiny fovea (see Figure 2) appears as a dimple in the very center of the macula. Densely packed with *only* cone cells, it is responsible for your most acute vision.

This process works flawlessly when your retina is healthy, and when there are no abnormalities in the front part of your eye. A normal eye sees the world in exquisite detail. Should any part of the eye fail, however, visual quality is lost.

Diseases of the Retina

IT IS important that you understand the meaning of the word "**disease.**" A disease is commonly misinterpreted as a condition that is contagious. That is true of some diseases, but not AMD. A disease is exactly what it says it is: a condition that causes "dis-ease," or an uncomfortable physical or mental state.[2] Specifically, AMD is a degenerative disease that results from aging, thus the name "age-related." It is but one (albeit the most common in seniors) of more than forty retinal diseases that can lead to visual impairment. There are over fifty forms of macular degeneration alone, which may help to explain the enormity of the task ahead.

You have very likely received an accurate diagnosis, but it is possible that your condition is better explained by another disease. It is also possible to have one or more retinal diseases simultaneously. If you think either of these is the case, do not hesitate to seek a second, or even third, opinion. Caring doctors will understand, and they may even recommend someone else to you. If you ask (in writing), your doctor will also send copies of your records to the new clinic.

Diseases of other parts of the eye are not included in this book, though several of them often afflict AMD patients. The most common are **cataracts, glaucoma, dry eye syndrome,** and certain **infections.** You will find definitions of those conditions in the glossary.

IN A SENTENCE:

> *By learning the terminology, you can communicate efficiently with your doctor and save valuable time in your appointments.*

learning

Visual Symptoms of AMD

FOCAL POINTS:

▶ *Learn to recognize what you are seeing.*
▶ *Learn to track your own visual changes.*

IF YOU are in the early stage of AMD, you probably haven't yet noticed any visual symptoms. Your doctor, however, probably sees drusen in your retina, swelling (edema), and/or discoloration of the retinal pigment epithelium (RPE). If you are in one of the later stages of AMD, you may be experiencing one or more of the following visual symptoms in addition to the scotomas and distortion discussed earlier:

Loss of color sensitivity. Some people with AMD gradually lose their color perception. This is because the photoreceptor cone cells, as discussed earlier, are responsible for color vision. The rod cells provide only black and shades of gray.[3]

Loss of acuity. Acuity refers to the level of clarity, distinction, or sharpness of your vision. Several eye charts have been devised to measure acuity. The most familiar of them, the **Snellen chart**, will be described in the "Living" section.

Floaters. Floaters are actually cellular debris within the vitreous fluid of the eye. You may see them as strings, streaks, clouds, bugs, dots, dust, or spider webs. They appear to be in front of your eye, but they are actually floating in the vitreous and casting shadows on your retina.

Floaters may interfere with reading and can be quite bothersome. There is no way to get rid of them aside from breaking them up with a laser or replacing the vitreous (a surgical procedure called a **vitrectomy**), but you can get used to them after a while.

For the most part, floaters are usually nothing to worry about, but they could signal a problem that requires treatment. While floaters may simply result from normal aging of the vitreous, they could be blood or torn retinal tissue. If new floaters appear, let your doctor know.

Light shows. The appearance of flashing, strobing, or waves of light is a very common symptom of AMD. Many patients experience these displays as the result of benign **posterior vitreous detachments (PVD)**, which can cause misfiring of the retinal nerve cells. Benign PVDs are not dangerous, and no surgery is required.

Another cause of light shows is the vitreous gel rubbing against or pulling on the retina. These flashing lights can be seen as sparkles, disco lights, fireflies, lightning, or fireworks. If you have ever been hit in the head and seen stars, you have witnessed what can happen when the retina is stimulated abnormally.

Light flashes are common during the aging process, and they are generally not cause for concern. If, however, a significant number of new floaters appears, accompanied by light flashes and partial sight loss (resembling a "curtain" blocking your vision), call your doctor immediately. These symptoms may indicate a **retinal tear** or **detachment**, damage that can be repaired successfully if caught in time.

Migraine flashers can also add to this personal light show. They appear as zigzag, shimmering, or even colorful lines that may move within the visual field. They usually last from five to thirty minutes and can occur in both eyes at once. They are most likely caused by a sudden spasm of blood vessels in the brain. These flashers are often associated with headache, nausea, or dizziness, but more often occur without such symptoms. In this case, they are commonly called an **ophthalmic migraine**, or a migraine without the other accompanying symptoms.

Double vision. This annoying condition is caused by one eye seeing differently than the other. As you read earlier, AMD is a **bilateral** disease; but the eyes do not lose vision equally. Swelling of the retinal tissues can cause distortion, throwing off the focal point of one eye. The problem then becomes which one to believe as they both fight for attention. A prism added to your spectacle prescription might take care of the problem by correcting the focal point of your "bad" eye. This is probably a temporary measure, however, as that eye is likely in a constant state of change. You may find yourself needing a new prescription more often.

Another solution is to cover the offending eye with a patch, or simply close it. Eventually, you will find that you won't notice the double vision as much, because your "good" eye will start to dominate, while your "bad" eye will become weaker from disuse. That's when double vision will be noticeable only on bright days, when the degenerating photoreceptors receive stronger stimulation. Sunglasses will help to alleviate the problem at that point.

Visual hallucinations. Some people report seeing images that are actually not there. Sometimes diagnosed as **Charles Bonnet Syndrome (CBS)**, it is thought to be the brain's way of trying to make up for lost input. CBS is not harmful, but it can be disconcerting at times. This **syndrome** is characterized by visual hallucinations in people who have significant loss of vision. It may be aggravated by other circumstances, such as sensory deprivation (as when living alone) and diminished cognitive abilities from stroke or aging.

It is important to keep in mind that CBS is not a psychotic condition and that it is not a serious mental illness. Most people who experience it report that their hallucinations are positive, and even pleasant, such as colorful flowers or dancing children. Friends and family members need to understand that this is a normal occurrence in many visually impaired people and that they should approach it with empathy and a good sense of humor. If, however, you experience hallucinations that are disturbing and persistent, consider scheduling an examination to eliminate the possibility of a neurological disorder or other physical pathology.

living

Monitor Your Own Vision

YOU SHOULD personally monitor your vision for two reasons: (1) to identify significant changes so you can notify your doctor, and (2) for your own peace of mind. You will feel better knowing where the enemy is at all times. Three self tests will be introduced here.

The Snellen chart

The most familiar eye test is the Snellen chart, named for its inventor, Dr. Hermann Snellen. People with 20/20 vision are considered to have normal acuity. If your acuity is such that you cannot see the largest letter on the chart (20/400 or worse), the doctor may have you stand closer or may hold up fingers for you to count. For lesser vision, hand motion or light perception tests may be used.[4] Figure 5 is the chart that most doctors use to determine your visual acuity. You can get an approximate measurement of your

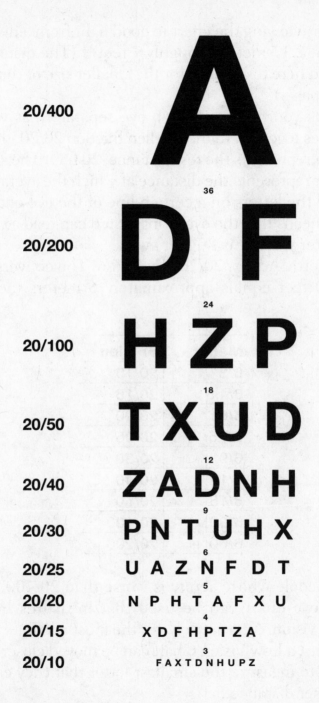

Figure 5. Snellen chart

acuity by viewing the chart in good light from a distance of about 2.17 meters (roughly 7 feet).[5] (The distance is adjusted here to account for the smaller size of the chart on the page.)

Check your acuity in each eye separately, as well as both eyes together. In the Snellen fraction 20/20, the first number represents the test distance, 20 feet. The second number represents the distance at which the average eye can see the letters on a certain line of the eye chart. So 20/20 means that the eye being tested can read a certain size letter when it is 20 feet away.

In Metric Acuity, 20/20 equals 6/6. The conversion is that 20 feet equals approximately 6 meters (actually 6.096).

Metric	Snellen
6/3	20/10
6/4.5	20/15
6/6	20/20
6/7.5	20/25
6/9	20/30
6/12	20/40
6/15	20/50
6/30	20/100
6/60	20/200

For people whose acuity is worse than 20/400, a different eye chart can be used that measures beyond 20/400 vision. Alternatively, for the most accurate measurements, a Low Vision Chart can be moved closer to the patient to measure the smallest letter that they can see at a lesser distance.

Vision worse than 20/400 can also be measured as Count Fingers (CF at a certain number of feet), Hand Motion (HM at a certain number of feet), Light Perception (LP), or No Light Perception (NLP). The conversion of Snellen Acuity to Count Fingers Acuity is as follows:

Snellen	Count Fingers
20/800	CF10'
20/1000	CF 8'
20/1143	CF 7'
20/1333	CF 6'
20/1600	CF 5'
20/2000	CF 4'
20/2666	CF 3'
20/4000	CF 2'
20/8000	CF 1'

Legal blindness is defined as having 20/200 best-corrected vision in the better eye or a visual field of less than 20 degrees. This standard was established in the United States *only* to help determine a person's eligibility for government benefits.

Legal blindness is not a measurement of your ability to function, and it does not mean that you are blind.

The Amsler grid

This test was probably one of the first introduced to you. It is a simple means of identifying changes in your vision and communicating them to your doctor. You can point out areas of distortion and blank spots in your central field, and you can even trace them directly onto the paper for your doctor to see. Several printed and electronic variations of the Amsler grid have been devised, but here is the basic version:

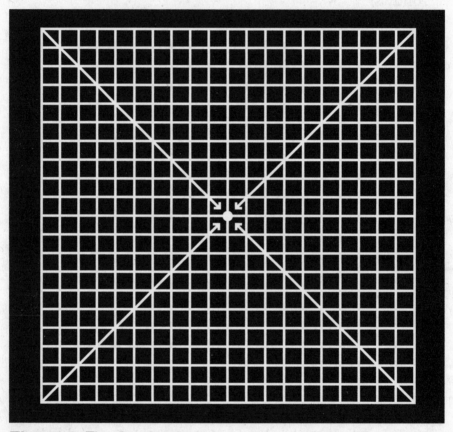

Figure 6. The Amsler grid

To accomplish the test, while wearing your reading glasses, hold this book approximately 18 inches from your face and close either eye. While fixing your gaze on the center of the grid, observe the surrounding area peripherally. If any lines are distorted ("bent"), this is evidence of swelling of your retina. Missing lines indicate either that fluid is blocking the light to your photo-receptor cells or that they are damaged. Use the Amsler grid regularly, and contact your doctor if you notice any significant and sudden changes.

The visual field grid

Your doctor has visual field testing devices in the clinic, but here is a simple way to map blind spots yourself (Figure 7). It is a variation of the Amsler grid designed specifically to identify scotomas. Before beginning, you may want to make copies of the grid.[6]

Turn the book so that the chart is upright. While gazing at the target in the center of the grid, close one eye and move the book toward your face until one of the oval spots disappears. (This is your **natural blind spot,** where the optic nerve enters the back of your eyeball. There are no photoreceptor cells in that area.) While continuing to focus on the target, make note of those squares in which the numbers are visible.

This is not an acuity test. You do not need to identify the numbers. They are there only for reference. Just take note of whether you can see that something white is in the square. If you are doing this alone, you may need to look away from the center in order to identify the numbers for recording purposes. If you have a helper, simply point to the squares and let your assistant write down the numbers for you. When all numbers have been listed, darken in those squares that were **not visible**. Then, using another copy of the grid, repeat the test for the other eye.

When you discuss your Amsler or Visual Field grids

with your doctor, it is important to know that the image you see on the paper is upside down and backwards from that which the doctor sees when he examines your retina. The lens in your eye inverts the image, just like the lens in a camera. Also, if you see something on a given side of your visual field, your doctor sees it on the other side. This is why the terms **nasal** (toward the nose) and **temporal** (toward the ear) are used, rather than "left" or "right."

Your doctor will be impressed and appreciative if you are familiar with some of the terminology. Better yet, you will be able to understand the language she uses. And don't worry about having to memorize it all. A complete glossary of ophthalmic terms and definitions may be found at the end of this book.

IN A SENTENCE:

> *The more you know about your symptoms, the better partner you can be with your doctor in your care and treatment.*

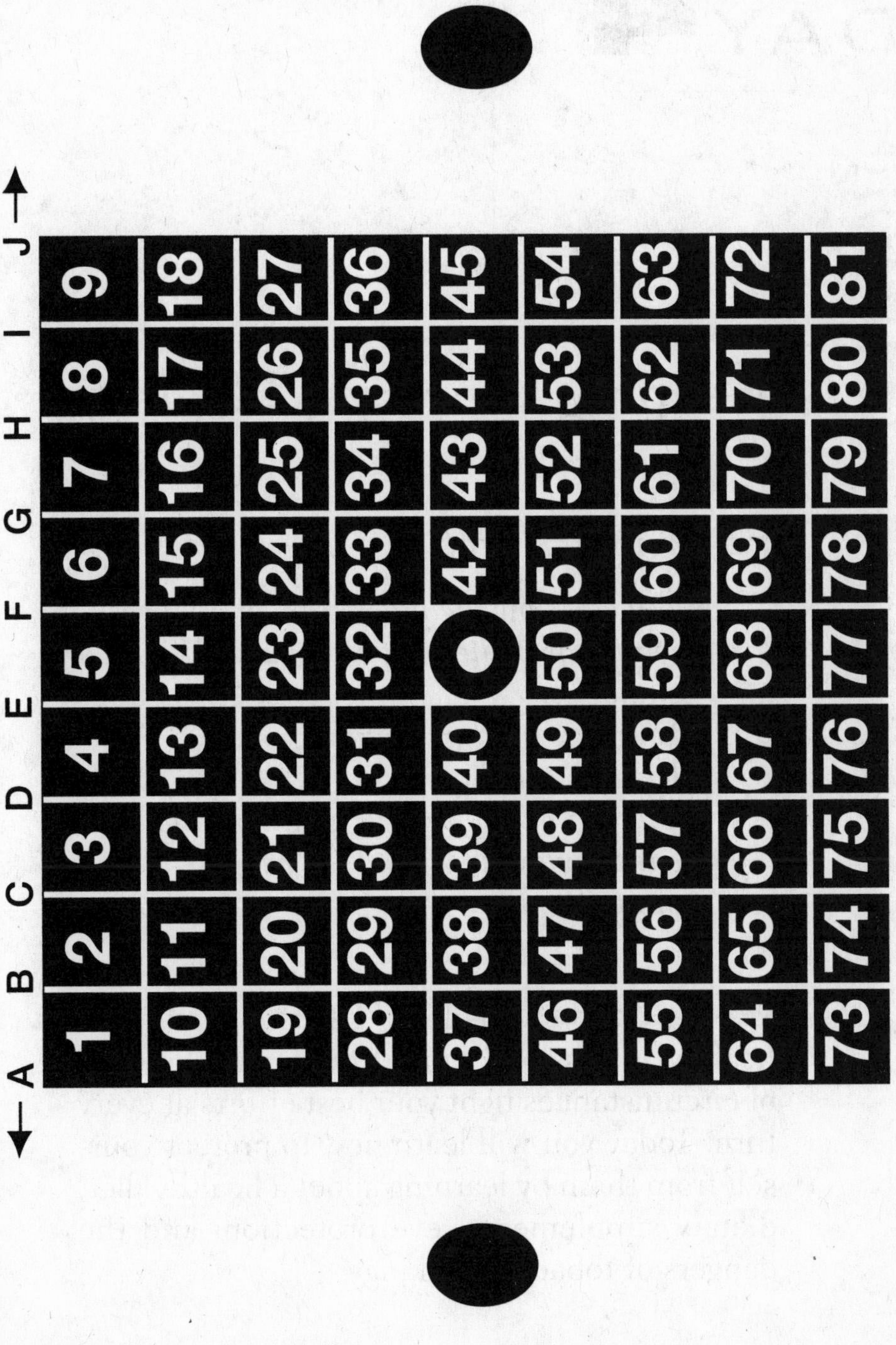

Figure 7. Visual Field Grid

DAY 4

learning

Keeping Your Eyes Healthy

FOCAL POINTS:

▶ *You can slow the progression of AMD with proven dietary and behavioral strategies.*

▶ *Your eyes need protection from hazardous light.*

▶ *You can maintain your quality of life by educating yourself and the people around you.*

WHAT CAN you do to keep your eyes as healthy as possible? Unfortunately, a whole set of circumstances fight your best efforts at every turn. Today you will learn how to protect yourself from them by learning about a healthy diet, dietary supplements, eye protection, and the dangers of tobacco smoking

Healthy diet

Your first and most controllable defense against AMD is a healthy diet. This means not only controlling *what* you eat, but also *how much* you eat. (Yes, obesity has been linked to AMD.[7, 8]) Since one of the biggest benefits of food comes from levels of antioxidants, an explanation of that process is covered here first.

Oxygen is important to the life of most of your cells. Internal **oxidation** is a chemical reaction produced by oxygen when energy is created from the food you digest. During this process, thousands of unbalanced electrons (**free radicals**) are released that can damage every cell in your body, including your eyes. Fortunately, **antioxidants** from particular foods and supplements supply the missing electrons required to balance the chaotic free radicals. All tissues are vulnerable to oxidative damage, but the most active tissues suffer the most, and that includes tissues in the retina and the brain.

It is important to remember that when free radical numbers increase past your natural defense system, the result can be disease and accelerated aging. Several circumstances can increase the number of free radicals. These are tobacco smoke, UV rays and blue light, pollution, alcohol, radiation, as well as physical and mental trauma. Such influences can be particularly controlled by healthy lifestyle choices and a diet of food containing large amounts of antioxidants.

While antioxidant vitamin supplements are good for you, be aware that the combination of the nutrients in food may have the greatest effect. Here are the top-ranking commonly eaten fruits and vegetables, listed from highest in antioxidant values to least.[9]

Fruits	Vegetables
Prunes	Kale
Raisins	Spinach
Blueberries	Brussels sprouts
Blackberries	Alfalfa sprouts
Strawberries	Broccoli flowers
Raspberries	Beets
Plums	Red bell pepper
Oranges	Onion
Red grapes	Corn
Cherries	Eggplant
Kiwi fruit	
Grapefruit, pink	

Recent research recommends adding to this diet at least three or four servings per week of coldwater fish for consumption of the important omega-3 fatty acids EPA and DHA.[10] Fish with the highest amount of omega-3 EPA/DHA are wild chinook or sockeye salmon, European anchovies, Atlantic or Pacific herring, small Atlantic or Pacific mackerel, black and red caviar, shrimp, and Pacific sardines.

Large ocean fish should be avoided or limited (such as halibut, grouper, and tuna) because of their excessively high mercury content. And caution should be taken when purchasing farm-raised salmon, which is now associated with excessively high amounts of omega-6 arachidonic acid. Omega-6 is already plentiful in your diet, and too much of it can lead to uncontrolled inflammation, which is thought to be a major cause of AMD.[11] For this very reason, Health and Welfare Canada recommends a 4 to 1 ratio of omega-6 to omega-3.[12] With this ratio, also recommended by the U.S. Institute of Medicine, the body can normally do a very good job of appropriately controlling the silent inflammatory process now thought to contribute to many diseases. Fish that contain dangerously high amounts of omega-6 are grouper, halibut, pompano, catfish, and Atlantic salmon. If you don't like fish, or just don't want to eat much of it, omega-3 can be obtained from freshly ground flaxseed or in stable, mercury-free fish oil supplements.

Now add to your retina-healthy diet ten or more servings of tomato products (preferably cooked) per week for lycopene and a handful of almonds daily for vitamin E. And don't forget zeaxanthin (zee-ah-ZAN'-thin) and lutein (LOO-teen). Research has found that the **carotenoids** lutein and zeaxanthin are strongly associated with reduced risk of AMD. A 1995 study showed that in addition to their value as antioxidants, lutein and zeaxanthin may help to protect the retina from long-term exposure to UV and blue light.[13] In effect, they act like sunglasses for AMD people who have lost the protective pigment (coloration) of their retinas. A 2004 study showed that lutein not only helps prevent AMD, it can actually reverse the symptoms.[14]

Neither of these nutritives is produced by your body. The necessary amount of lutein, for example, must be acquired from five to nine servings a day of fruits and vegetables.[15] Since this amount is difficult to achieve for most people, doctors recommend that the slack be taken up by supplements.

A 2003 study found that zeaxanthin is the dominant component in the center of the macula, while lutein dominates at the outer edges.[16] This distribution of lutein and zeaxanthin may indicate that they have different functions, with zeaxanthin being more critical. A high level of zeaxanthin might, therefore, be important for best protection. Dosages of up to 10 milligrams are included in commercially available dietary supplements and can also be purchased separately. No recommended daily allowances have been established, but most nutritionists recommend daily amounts of 20 milligrams of lutein and 10 milligrams of zeaxanthin.

Foods that are high in zeaxanthin (listed from most to least) are:

Eggs
Pepper, orange (raw)
Corn, sweet, yellow (canned)
Persimmons, Japanese (raw)
Corn, frozen (cooked)
Spinach (raw)
Turnip greens (cooked)
Collard greens (cooked)
Lettuce, cos or romaine (raw)
Spinach (cooked)
Kale (cooked)
Tangerine, mandarin[17]

Foods that are high in lutein (again listed from most to least) are:

Kale (raw)
Kale (cooked)
Spinach (cooked)
Collards (cooked)
Turnip greens (cooked)
Spinach (fresh, raw)

Broccoli (cooked)
Romaine lettuce (raw)
Green peas (canned)
Corn (canned)
Corn (cooked)
Green beans (cooked)
Eggs (raw)
Orange juice (frozen, from concentrate)
Orange (raw)
Papaya (raw)
Tangerine (raw)[18]

A diet that includes five to nine servings a day of the above foods should provide nearly everything healthy eyes need for good vision. Unfortunately, people with AMD are not blessed with healthy eyes, so you may need extra help in the form of dietary supplements as outlined earlier.

Dosages in supplements are based upon the assumption that you eat well. They are called supplements because they are meant to enhance your normal diet, not to replace it. If you can establish exceptionally good eating habits, the only additional nutrients your eyes may need are those powerhouse antioxidants that are difficult to ingest in sufficient quantities. At the top of the list are vitamin E, alpha-lipoic acid, CoQ10, and acetyl-L-carnitine. Anthocyanidins (from very dark berries) are also important, as they have been shown to control chronic inflammation and stabilize vascular endothelial growth factor (VEGF). VEGF, as discussed in Week 2, has been associated with AMD. Sufficient amounts of the B-complex vitamins can be difficult to obtain from your normal diet. Therefore, you probably need to supplement in order to control any possibility of your body producing excessive amounts of homocystine, which can be associated with AMD retinal bleeds.

As another example, almonds are a good source of vitamin E, but they are high in calories and fats. Therefore, you would not want to eat enough of them to acquire the recommended 400 IU (International Units) per day. If you don't get it in other foods, then that is when vitamin E supplementation becomes important. And here is good news for chocolate lovers. Wine and green tea have been known for a while to be high-antioxidant drinks, but now hot cocoa has been added to the recommended list. Cocoa has almost twice the antioxidant power of wine and two to three times that of green tea, according to a 2003 study.[19] Chocolate candy is also a source of antioxidants, but then you are adding calories, as well. Remember what your grandmother always told you: moderation in all things is best (and that goes for wine, too).

Each person's body metabolizes food differently, which makes generalizations difficult, just as nutrient intake from food sources is not always dependable, based on growing conditions and time from harvest to table. Fortunately, your body will usually tell you what you need, so pay attention to it. By the time your eyes tell you, however, it may be too late to reverse the damage. Nutritional scientists strongly recommend taking daily biochemically balanced multivitamins that cover the full range of nutrients instead of a little of this and a little of that. Micronutrient balance is vitally important, and it's easy to take too much of one vitamin or mineral and not enough of another when you are taking many different supplements. This, again, is a good reason to work with your eye care specialist, your general physician, and a qualified nutritionist to create the dietary plan that works best for you. Your effort could pay off in extra years of good health and vision.

Dietary supplements

Dietary supplements are nutrients that come in tablet or liquid form. Supplements may help if you are unable to ingest the necessary quantities of antioxidants. Just be careful that you do not overdose on vitamins that are fat soluble, as they can be toxic. The fat-soluble vitamins to be wary of are **beta-carotene** (a precursor of vitamin A) and vitamins D, E, and K. Keep in mind, however, that vitamin D allows your body to absorb enough calcium for strong bones. It is also important protection against muscle weakness and possibly against the risk of breast, prostrate, and colon cancer. Vitamin D should not be eliminated entirely, but either 400 to 600 IU daily or brief periods of exposure to sunlight (your skin, not your eyes) will satisfy your requirement. Vitamin E (tocopherols) is also important to general health, so 400 IU daily is a reasonable and safe dosage.

Antioxidant supplements that are water soluble are safe in reasonable amounts, because your body will eliminate excess dosages. These are vitamin C and the B vitamins including folic acid. The folic acid/B vitamin/ homocysteine issue is important for general health, including eye health, and recent studies suggest a connection between elevated homocysteine level and wet AMD.

Antioxidants in the form of vitamins are the most common nutrients for AMD. Here is an introduction to those that are most important:

The AREDS formula (supplements for early-stage AMD)

In the late 1990s the **Age-Related Eye Disease Study (AREDS)**, funded by the National Eye Institute, concluded that certain dosages of antioxidant vitamins and zinc would help preserve vision and moderately lower the risk of developing wet AMD.[20] Many vitamin companies are now manufacturing supplements containing variations of the dosages used in the study. The AREDS-recommended dosages are: vitamin C, 500 milligrams; vitamin E, 400 IU; beta-carotene, 15 milligrams; and zinc, 80 milligrams. It is important to remember that the science behind the AREDS formulation is from 1988. Other studies of other nutrients published in peer-reviewed literature strongly suggest including other nutrients in the daily supplements of AMD patients, as well as for those people with high familial risk factors for AMD.

Modifications to the AREDS formula have been made by some companies, such as lowering dosages of zinc and increasing the amount of copper. Some formulas have eliminated beta-carotene for patients who smoke. Some companies have included the AREDS formula with a cocktail of other vitamins and nutrients to satisfy recommended daily requirements and to bolster retinal health with other ingredients reputed to be beneficial. Most recognized brand names that follow the AREDS formula are Bi-Sight, Macula Complete, Ocuvite Preservision, SightMart, VisiVite, VitEyes, and Vision-Nutrition. Some are available only online, so ask for them by name at your local store.

If you take the AREDS formula, you should not also take a full multisupplement. Multisupplements contain the ingredients in the AREDS formula, so you do not want to risk overdosing. Either purchase extra nutrients separately (which can get confusing and expensive), or purchase them from a company that includes essential nutrients in the same tablet or capsule as the AREDS formula. If you shop around, you will find what you need, but remember, it is *very important* that you consult with your eye care specialist *and* your general physician before making significant changes in your diet or nutrition supplements.

The AREDS researchers found that patients with advanced cases of dry AMD or vision loss due to wet AMD in one eye had a significantly lower chance of developing wet AMD when taking the AREDS formula. If you have wet AMD, however, you should be cautious about taking the formula (which contains 400 IU of vitamin E, a blood thinner) along with blood-thinning agents for arthritis or cardiovascular problems. Again, it is essential that you discuss this with your eye care specialist and your general physician.

A second AREDS study is under way to reexamine the original dosages and to study potential benefits of nutrients not included in the original formula. Those nutrients include lutein, zeaxanthin, and omega-3 fatty acids. Combinations of those nutrients will also be looked at in the study.

Other studies

Two other important studies are worth mentioning here. One out of Italy found no disease progression and reduced amounts of drusen in the eyes of diagnosed AMD patients who took a supplement that included acetyl-L-carnitine, CoQ10, and omega-3 EPA/DHA. This particular combination of nutrients has also been studied for years by Bruce Ames, PhD, biochemist at the University of California–Berkeley.[21]

Another study found a 35 percent reduction in the risk of AMD in those people who ate a very well-balanced diet with foods that contained a high amount of antioxidants, including those in the AREDS formula. This is important because the original AREDS found no reduction in the risk of AMD in those patients who simply took the AREDS formulation. In addition, the researchers established only a 25 percent reduction in the progression of AMD. Obviously, you need *both* a healthy diet *and* a well-designed program of supplementation to target the specific causes of cellular injury associated with AMD.

Eye protection and light hazards

Excessively bright sunlight can be harmful to your eyes. A wide-brimmed hat and wraparound sunglasses that filter UV and blue light are your best protection against the sun's **ultraviolet (UV)** rays and hazardous visible light. **Polarization** is also helpful, as that process filters out horizontal glare (from water surfaces or wet roads).

The lenses of sunglasses that block 100 percent **blue light** (wavelengths from 400 to 500 nanometers) are tinted orange or amber. Any other tint is letting part of the blue light spectrum through. You should not, however, drive with 100 percent "blue blockers," as they change your color perception. School buses and yellow road stripes, for example, will appear pink. And don't worry if your color perception is out of kilter for a while after removing the glasses. Your brain just needs time to reprogram itself.

And now let's talk about the problems that can arise from the wrong kind of artificial lighting in your home or workplace.

Sight requires light. On the other hand, the wrong kind and intensity of light can destroy sight. As years go by, your retinas grow more sensitive to damage from chronic light exposure.[22, 23, 24] According to some studies, blue light waves may be especially toxic to retinas that are prone to AMD.[25, 26] Whereas the shorter UV wavelengths are somewhat filtered by the lens and cornea, studies of animal and human retinal cells have shown that the light spectrum from UV through blue can be harmful. Experiments on both animal and human retinal cells have shown that as the wavelengths grow shorter, toxicity (poisoning) of the retina increases.[27, 28]

Fortunately, healthy retinas have a wide array of built-in chemical defenses against UV and blue light damage. These defenses bear such imposing names as xanthophyll, **melanin,** superoxide dismutase, catalase, and glutathione peroxidase. And then there are the more familiar agents: vitamin E, vitamin C, lutein, and zeaxanthin. Unfortunately, these defenses can weaken with disease, injury, neglect, and age, so, as we discussed earlier, dietary supplements may help.

Another built-in protective process occurs as your natural lens take on a yellowish tint over the years, helping to filter blue light.[29, 30] After cataract surgery, however, patients lose that benefit. Some doctors now recommend replacing the damaged lens with a yellow-tinted **intraocular lens (IOL)**.[31] This may help, but be aware that a tinted IOL will somewhat diminish night vision.[32]

Blue light is an important element in "natural" lighting, and it may also contribute to psychological health. You will find over twenty different brands of so-called full-spectrum, or daylight, task lamps on the market. Most of them advertise that they promote good vision, because they imitate sunshine. Your doctor, if unaware of the research, might even recommend that you purchase one. Think twice, however. If your doctor says the sun is bad for your eyes, why would you want to bring sunlight indoors and place it on your desktop?

We need bright lighting, but lamps that replicate sunshine might not only hasten our sight loss, they can also cause significant discomfort. When you read outdoors, would you rather sit in the direct sun or in the shade? Which provides the best light to read by? The shade is the more comfortable, of course, and even more so when supplemented by a good pair of sunglasses. Sunlight, obviously, is not the light you want.

What kind of artificial lighting should a person with AMD use? As discussed above, a good amount of research shows that prolonged exposure to light containing peak levels of blue wavelengths (close to ultraviolet) can be harmful. One study even suggests that the lower the intensity of blue light, the faster the reading rate of AMD patients.[33]

A study of the Chesapeake Bay watermen also reported a significant association between blue light and age-related macular degeneration.[34, 35] In view of this kind of scientifically based evidence, people who are at risk for retinal degeneration should avoid high-intensity light sources with a color temperature of 5000 degrees K (Kelvin) or higher. This is the intensity of blue light on a bright sunny day at noon. Nearly every full-spectrum or daylight lamp on the market falls into this potentially hazardous range.[36]

The safest and brightest task lamps that also provide the best contrast and economy of operation are *white halogen* and *warm-colored fluorescent* types. Specify this when you purchase, and be sure to also specify a color temperature of *less than 5000 degrees K*.[37] If the salesperson doesn't understand what you mean, try another store. And remember, regular incandescent lightbulbs are very safe, even at high wattage, if you don't mind the cost of using them and the slight loss of contrast from their yellowish output.

Remember, research is showing that high levels of exposure to blue or visible light may cause ocular damage, especially later in life, and may be related to the development of age-related macular degeneration.[38] These findings, even though not conclusive, should motivate you to be cautious about the kind of lighting you use.

Avoidance of tobacco smoking

A link between smoking and AMD has long been known.[39] Tobacco smoking lowers the density of pigment in the retina, which decreases the protection it offers from harmful light. As a result, smokers have two to four times the risk of developing macular degeneration,[40, 41, 42] and the effects of smoking last for up to twenty years. The quantity of cigarettes smoked can make a difference in the amount of risk.[43]

You may hear that your risk of developing lung cancer increases if you smoke and take beta-carotene. This information came from the "Physicians' Health Study" in 1995,[44] which resulted in many **nutraceutical** companies removing beta-carotene from recommended antioxidant formulas. Not all studies, however, have shown that risk. One study even concluded that the risk of lung cancer in smokers actually *declines* as a result of taking beta-carotene *when taken in combination with other supplements.*[45] Along this same line, there is no evidence to suggest that smokers should cut down on foods with high levels of beta-carotene.

The body converts beta-carotene to vitamin A, and vitamin A is essential to good vision.[46] If your only reason for not taking beta-carotene is that you smoke, then why not stop smoking? That is decidedly difficult, but you (and the people around you) will benefit in more ways than one. This has been a day full of important information for maintaining your visual health. The major points are listed here for your review:

Focus on the Facts

Extra-body circumstances that can harm your retinas are tobacco smoke, UV rays and blue light, pollution, alcohol, radiation, physical trauma, and illness.

Excessively bright sunlight can be harmful to your eyes.

Blue light may be especially toxic to retinas that are prone to AMD.

You can help to protect your retinas from oxidation by eating a healthy diet, protecting your eyes, avoiding tobacco smoking, and taking nutritional supplements as recommended by your doctor.

Work with your eye care specialist, your general physician, and a qualified nutritionist to create the dietary plan that works best for you.

living

Your Life:
Quality vs. Quantity

DAY 4 has focused on steps you can take to slow vision loss from AMD. If you succeed in doing so, your quality of life will increase.

At the same time, your doctors, family members, and friends may be greatly underestimating the impact AMD has on you as the patient. AMD inhibits living activities and pleasures that you have gotten used to over many years. You should be enjoying the fruits of a life of labor and learning, not having to start this unexpected new life as a visually-impaired person. That can be devastating to you, and it can be worse when the people in your support system do not seem to understand.

A revealing study has drawn some interesting conclusions related to this issue. The researchers endeavored to "assess individual preferences under situations of uncertainty . . . and determine whether members of the general public and clinicians could appreciate the impact that [AMD] can have on quality of well-being."[47] A questionnaire was distributed to 115 AMD patients. The essence of the questionnaire was to determine the number of years of life patients would be willing to trade for a permanent cure. The same questionnaire was distributed to healthy volunteers and clinicians in the field of low vision, all of whom were asked to assume they had AMD.

If you are an AMD patient yourself, the responses will probably not surprise you.[48] Patients with mild AMD would forgo an average of 61 days of one additional year of life if they could live the remainder of that year free of the disease. By comparison, the general public would forgo 15 days, and clinicians would forgo 26 days. Patients with moderate AMD would forgo an average of 98 days. By comparison, the general public would forgo 30 days, and clinicians would forgo 45 days. Patients with severe AMD would forgo an average of 158 days. By comparison, the general public would forgo 52 days, and clinicians would forgo 65 days.

These results revealed that the general public and clinicians considerably underestimated the impact that mild, moderate, and severe AMD has on a person's quality of well-being. The only two conditions for which patients were willing to trade a greater amount of time were total blindness and a severe brain disease that includes both physical and visual impairment.[49] The researchers' suppositions, quoted verbatim here, are provocative:

1. Members of the general public may not fully understand or appreciate that AMD ["MD" in the original text] causes blurring and distortion of central vision.
2. They may not take into consideration the numerous limitations resulting from decreased visual acuity such as difficulty in reading, driving, or performing activities of daily living without assistance.
3. The public probably does not appreciate the cost of frequent visits to the ophthalmologist and low vision aids, the increased risk of sustaining additional injuries such as hip fractures from accidents attributed to poor vision, or the anxiety of not knowing if or when the dry form of AMD may convert to the wet form, resulting in rapid loss of remaining vision.
4. Clinicians may not fully appreciate the consequences of vision loss. Alternatively, this group may have confidence that in the near future there will be effective therapies.[50]

This enlightening information dramatizes the need for better education of the people in your support system. Hopefully, they are also reading this book for a better understanding of the situation in which you have found yourself.

Living as a VIP in a sighted world

Most people are born with working retinas. If an infant's retinas are healthy and her eyes are in good condition, she soon becomes a visual learner. Eighty percent of her sensory input is received through her eyes, and nearly half of her brain is dedicated to interpreting the signals they send. Therefore, the infant's sense of sight becomes the center of almost everything she does—the center of her life, if you will.

If, on the other hand, she is severely myopic, or if her eyes are diseased, her brain will grow to depend less upon light input and more on her other senses. Her learning then becomes more dependent upon touch, smell, hearing, and taste. She also might find that her memory skills and creative intellect are elevated. In spite of her vision difficulties, she can still develop into a totally capable adult with the help of corrective lenses and/or low vision technology.

What happens, however, if she is fortunate enough to have healthy eyes early on, becomes visually dependent, and then develops late-stage AMD in the fifth or sixth decade of her life? She is still visually oriented in a visual world, but she has been robbed of her modus operandi. She is simply no longer equipped to live well in her own world. She realizes that humankind has created an environment that conveniences the majority: traffic lights, stairways, photographs, the printed word. No longer able to use her eyesight as well as before, she has lost a necessary part of herself. This is much like experiencing the death of a loved one. In some ways, it is worse. When death occurs, others can share the experience and the sorrow. AMD cannot be easily shared. Loss of eyesight is a personal and often lonely experience, because few people can truly identify with it.

Okay, so most people cannot really understand how you see or feel. They can, however, do their best to help. That is why electronic birds chirp at crosswalks and why ramps replace stairways. That is why companies produce descriptive movies, audiobooks, Braille, computer technology, personal satellite guidance systems, talking appliances, and even gadgets that beep at you when your teacup is full. Those things help you to get through the day more easily, which in turn lifts your spirit. And spirit can help you deal with the other aspects of your life.

The best approach, then, to living as a visually impaired person in a visual world is to learn how. Imagine yourself as an infant again. Train your other senses as you would have done if you had been born this way in the first place. It won't take as long as before, because this time you have years of wisdom and experience to draw upon. The following days, weeks, and months will provide additional guidance on how to live well with macular degeneration.

IN A SENTENCE:

> *You can help to maintain your quality of life through continuing education about proven strategies for the best physical and mental health.*

learning

A Journey through Low Vision Rehabilitation: Jim's Story

FOCAL POINTS:

- ◗ *Low vision technology will help maintain your quality of life.*
- ◗ *Low vision rehabilitation training will help you adapt.*

How it began

I noticed it after my last class on a Friday. While writing my history students' assignment on the board, I got some chalk in my right eye. I closed it for a second and couldn't see the letters I'd just written. I actually thought I'd accidentally erased them. That's what it looked like. Like I'd smudged them out with my hand or something. Then I opened my other eye, and the letters were there again.

I thought maybe there was a smear on my glasses, so I took them off. But that smudge was still there, right in the middle of my left eye. And when I looked at the frame around the board, it was all out of shape . . . distorted. I don't know why I hadn't noticed it before. I couldn't blink that spot away, or rub it away, or anything. It was just there, and I didn't know what was happening.

I was supposed to attend a staff meeting that afternoon, but I didn't. I just left. I had to find out what was going on, so I went straight home and called my optometrist. He made time for me that afternoon. To make a long story short, I knew in a few hours that I had an eye disease I had never heard of and couldn't even pronounce. I had become one of the visually impaired, and I was off on a trip I had never in my life expected to take.

Follow me as I retrace that journey, and I'll show you how a program of low vision rehabilitation training can help you to live successfully with sight loss. My hope is that by having this information early on, you will not have to experience the emotional distress and sense of helplessness that I did when I first faced a future with vision impairment.

What did I need?

My eye care specialist told me that vision impairment is generally any interference with sight that hinders the performance of daily activities. It can be caused by disease, trauma, or a congenital disorder, and it may appear as one or more of six general conditions:

Blurriness, where visual acuity with best spectacle correction is still reduced or blurred

Narrowing of peripheral or side vision

Defects within the field of vision, such as distortion or blind spots

Loss of contrast

Sensitivity to glare or light

Loss of color perception

The term **visually impaired** should not be confused with the term **legally blind**. I learned that legal blindness is defined as acuity of 20/200 or worse in the better eye with correction, or a visual field of 20 degrees or less in the better eye.

A person who meets one of these criteria might still have usable vision, but he would not be able to read without training on an assistive device. Also, he would not be able to meet the requirements for obtaining a driver's license. This person would be described as visually impaired, but another person who is visually impaired may not necessarily be legally blind.

So what is low vision rehabilitation? Well, for me it was like physical therapy if I had lost a limb. The purpose was to develop strategies to maximize or substitute for my diminished sight so that I could maintain my independence and sense of self-worth. This rebuilding and reinforcement of the visual foundation is mainly accomplished through identification of goals, introduction to low vision devices, and training.

My program was designed to provide education, support, and individual counseling. It also helped me to realize that using such devices and techniques is a sign of tenacity and courage, not weakness or defeat.

Vision rehabilitation specialists teach how to manage daily activities such as:

adapting the home for safety and navigation
improving lighting conditions
preparing meals
personal grooming
using magnifiers for easier reading
writing
labeling medications, clothing, and appliances
keeping financial records
systematizing shopping and payment at the register

I had some good reasons for entering low vision rehabilitation training. When my right eye went bad, I couldn't read, and I couldn't drive. I couldn't work in my woodshop, which bothered me a lot. I thought I was going totally blind. I became very depressed and decided that life as I had known it was pretty much over.

There was more stress at home. My family couldn't accept the fact that I didn't see well, and I just couldn't help out, couldn't do the carpentry, and couldn't help my kids build their houses. My wife, Marie, was very understanding, but it was difficult for her. I tried to continue teaching. The students and staff were very supportive in the beginning, but they seemed to forget after a while. Writing lesson plans and grading papers was difficult. I particularly had problems with reading textbooks and journals. So, with Marie's encouragement, I took the first big step by talking to my eye doctor about it, and I was on my way.

A **low vision therapist** called me and asked me questions about my health, eye condition, and my visual goals, things I wanted to do but couldn't because of my impairment. She explained how I could make the best use of my remaining sight through training, low vision devices, and services. Then I answered a lot of questions and took tests so she could determine how I was functioning and what my needs might be. I thought the questions would never end, but I knew how important they were. The rehab therapist didn't leave any stones unturned, that's for sure. I think that by the time she was through, she probably knew more about me than my own wife did, and after thirty-six years of marriage, that's saying a lot.

How was my vision?

The next step was a thorough exam by a **low vision specialist.** In addition to acuity tests, similar to the Snellen chart but specially designed for low vision patients, the doctor used four other tests:

> an **Amsler grid** to identify defects in my central visual field. (**Scanning laser ophthalmoscopy [SLO]** is also a good tool for mapping scotomas, but the cost of the instrument is high and not yet accessible to most doctors.)
>
> a **contrast sensitivity test** to determine my ability to discriminate subtle changes in vision that occur in the real world
>
> a **brightness acuity tester (BAT)** to look at the impact of glare on my retina
>
> a **color vision test** to check my color perception

My **ocular motility** was also evaluated to see if I had any impaired eye movement. And finally, I was given an external eye health evaluation, an intraocular pressure test, and an internal ocular examination. All of this confirmed that I was someone who would benefit from low vision rehabilitation training. And so I began.

How could I make daily living easier?

My training included safe cooking strategies, labeling techniques, use of adaptive equipment, and an evaluation of the safety and lighting in my home. Most of the training took place in a specially designed apartment at the center. I relearned everything. Things I had been doing my whole life I had to learn to do all over again, this time without depending so much on my eyesight. It wasn't easy. I trained twice a week for six weeks, and each session lasted for one or two hours.

My condition was not severe enough to require **orientation and mobility (O and M)** training. A person with nearly total vision loss would require about twenty-five hours of individualized sessions by an O and M specialist, with advanced training in actual public situations. The activity would also include several hours of calisthenics and walking. Skills such as safe street crossings, negotiating stairs and curbs, and utilizing public transportation would be learned, in addition to familiarization with new environments. Use of an animal guide would also be an important consideration, as would training in **Braille**.

An important part of my training was personal and marital counseling to help my family and me deal with my loss of vision. Gradually, my self-esteem and my confidence in my ability to overcome my vision impairment greatly improved.

The Three Bs for better vision— Bigger, Brighter, and Bolder

Another important part of my rehabilitation was training in low vision management. This dealt with modification of my environment and learning about low vision devices. The "Three B's" were considered when it came to maximizing my vision:

"Bigger": Magnification
"Brighter": Illumination
"Bolder": Contrast

When it came to learning about magnification devices, I was amazed at the variety of low vision gadgets and computer software that could help me. I was given hands-on experience with almost every kind of device imaginable. These included:

- prescription magnification or microscopic glasses
- a little telescope for reading street signs, identifying people, and seeing the sights
- computer software that magnifies my monitor screen and cursor
- magnification devices for my desktop and pocket

Descriptions of Low Vision Magnifiers

Handheld magnifier: "Sherlock Holmes" type portable magnifying glass. Clamps with flexible arms are available for attaching to tabletops.

Pros: Small and inexpensive. Available in a wide range of powers (1.5X–8X). Socially accepted.

Cons: Leaves only one hand free. Difficult to keep in focus if hand trembles.

Illuminated handheld magnifier: Portable lens with handle and built-in battery-operated light. Clamps with flexible arms are available for attaching to tabletops.

Pros: Small and inexpensive. Available in a wide range of powers (1.5X–8X). Socially accepted. Useful for viewing dimly lit areas.

Cons: Leaves only one hand free. Difficult to keep in focus if hand trembles.

Stand magnifier: Magnifier on a stand with built-in legs for tabletops or books.

Pros: Maintains steady focal distance. Comes in a wide range of powers (1.7X–8X). Possible to write beneath and use both hands.

Cons: Bulkier than handheld device. Sometimes difficult to get sufficient light between the lens and the subject.

Hand/Stand magnifier: Combination of handheld and stand magnifier.

Pros: Can be used as either by folding handle and legs, so more portable than a regular stand magnifier. Comes in powers of 2.5X–3X).

Cons: None.

Illuminated stand magnifier: Illuminated magnifier on a stand with built-in legs for tabletops or books. Light source is either a built-in battery-operated bulb, a halogen lamp (A/C), or LED illumination (D/C).

Pros: Provides shadowless light close to the subject. Maintains steady focal distance. Comes in a wide range of powers (1.7X–8X).

Cons: Difficult to write beneath most models. Even bulkier than an ordinary stand magnifier. Battery-operated models (except LED version) can be expensive to run.

Illuminated bench magnifier: Same as above, but mounted on an adjustable arm mounted to a tabletop or workbench.

Pros: Good for using both hands for sewing, hobbies, etc.

Cons: Limited magnification (rarely above 3X). Comparatively expensive.

Dome/Bright Field magnifier: Half-spherical magnifier (like a paperweight) that rests directly on the page. Largest dome available is 90mm.

Pros: Always in focus. Distributes light well onto the surface.

Cons: Made of heavy glass rather than plastic.

Bar magnifier: Semicylindrical lens that rests directly on the page, magnifying one line of print at a time.

Pros: Makes tracking of a line of text easier.

Cons: Limited level of magnification power (up to 3X). Reflected light and distortion can be problematic.

Spectacle-mounted magnifier: Magnification lenses mounted on spectacles. Single magnifying lenses (for one eye only) are available from 4X to 12X.

Pros: Leaves both hands free.

Cons: Short working distance due to limited level of magnification power of up to 3X.

Clip-on magnifier: Magnifying lens that attaches to regular spectacles. Binocular versions are available in powers 2X–4X. Monocular versions are available up to 7X.

Pros: Leaves both hands free.

Cons: Short working distance due to limited level of magnification power.

Handheld or spectacle-mounted telescope: Telescopes of low magnification (up to 4X) that can be mounted on spectacles for near intermediate and distance viewing.

Pros: Good for reading music, viewing TV or plays, reading signs, etc.

Cons: Restricted field of view. Best for stationary viewing. Focus is automatic or fixed, depending upon model.

Field expanders/minifiers: Lenses that reduce the apparent size of the subject (like a peephole in a door).

Pros: Useful for people with good central vision but diminished peripheral vision.

Cons: None.

Closed-circuit television (CCTV)/video magnifier: Device utilizing a camera and monitor to magnify a page or object. The display can be monochrome or full color, and the products are available in a variety of screen sizes and magnification levels. Some models are designed for interconnection with computers.

Pros: Books and objects can be placed beneath the camera for viewing. Sufficient room to write.

Cons: Comparatively expensive. Not portable.

Portable (CCTV)/video magnifier: Portable magnifying device utilizing a camera approximately the size of a computer mouse, plus an interface for connecting to a standard television or head-mounted display. Battery power optional.

Pros: Can be carried in a purse or backpack. Less expensive than stationary CCTV models.

Cons: Some practice required for smooth operation of the handheld camera. One-handed operation. Cannot be used for magnification of writing or handwork.

The rehabilitation specialists also showed me **non-optical devices** available from stores and catalogs, including:

    bold-tipped pens
    large-print books and magazines
    talking books
    check-writing guides
    talking watches, clocks, and scales
    lighting instruments
    book holders
    an electronic scanner that reads books to me

My rehab team figured out exactly what I needed to see better and to live an almost normal life again. Marie and the kids went shopping out of one of those catalogs for my birthday, and I actually use everything I got. Even stuff I didn't know I needed, like a gadget that tells me when my cup is getting full so that I don't pour coffee all over the table. I can't wait until Christmas now.

My low vision therapist taught me that **illumination** is probably the most important aspect of my environment. It is also the easiest to modify. Because of my vision impairment, I needed more light than normal. So we increased the number of lamp fixtures and made sure to use only the safest lighting for my retinas.

For general lighting, we installed regular incandescent floodlights and walkway lights on the outside of the house. For near-vision tasks, we placed white halogen lighting at my desk and reading chair. We also made certain that all fluorescent lighting used "warm fluorescent lamps."

Next, we identified and eliminated all potential sources of **glare** by adding window shades, securing scatter rugs on the polished wood floor in the dining room, and making a cutout line guide for reading magazines with glossy pages. I also keep my brimmed hat and my *tinted* and *polarized* glasses handy for any other situations that might occur, either indoors or out.

Contrast is also very important to good vision, so with the help of my therapist, my wife and I:

- ○ installed faceplates on electrical switches and outlets in contrasting color to the wall
- ○ covered a glass-topped table with a dark-colored tablecloth
- ○ applied dark-colored decals to a sliding glass door
- ○ laid a dark-colored bath mat over the edge of the tub
- ○ placed a rubber ball in the bathtub to help me see the water level
- ○ wrapped rings of bright tape around handles of pots, tools, and utensils
- ○ labeled my computer's keys with white-on-black stickers (they make black-on-white, too)
- ○ attached a filter to my computer monitor to reduce glare
- ○ applied white paint to the leading edge of our porch steps
- ○ painted my work table a solid, nonglossy tan to reduce what my therapist called "figure-ground clutter" and allow me to find my tools more easily

The therapist complimented me on already having my tools fairly well organized on pegboards, and smaller items, such as nails and screws, separated into drawers. I had to admit, that was Marie's doing.

Where can you get low vision rehabilitation training?

I was fortunate to have an outstanding rehabilitation center near my home. You can find one by asking your doctor, contacting your state agency (see Appendix A) or calling the American Optometric Association at (415) 561-8540. If you have access to the Internet, another excellent online resource is the search tool at www.vision-connection.com.

If you don't meet the eligibility requirements of your state blindness agency, but your employment is being adversely affected, you can go for help to the state's vocational rehabilitation agency (also listed in Appendix A).

The referral mechanism differs slightly with each state, but generally, you can request training, or you can be referred by a family member, a friend, your eye care specialist, or a social worker. State statutes specify the minimum levels of vision loss for entry into the program, but there is also some flexibility in the acceptance standards.

State agencies will usually cover the costs of rehabilitation for people who are registered. If you have not qualified for government assistance, you should expect to pay your own expenses.

How am I doing now?

Since my initial low vision assessment and training, I have greatly improved my skills for independent functioning. Vision rehabilitation isn't easy, and it isn't a cure for blindness. It's an educational process that requires patience, practice, flexibility, and motivation. As I always told my students, if a person doesn't have a real reason to want to learn—a ton of self-motivation—then there isn't anyone who is going to be able to teach them.

It was a long road, but I don't even want to think how long the rest of this road would be without the confidence and independence those people have given me. They gave me the tools, taught me how to use them, and showed me that my life can be just as good as it always was. Different, maybe—not the way I thought it was going to be—but it's good.

living

Acceptance Doesn't Mean Giving In

"WHY DO you people always talk about accepting macular degeneration? I will never accept what is happening to my eyes! If you want to just lie down and die, then go ahead. But you'll do it without me."

With that, M. J. left the support group and never returned. Having been with the group for only a week, she misconstrued the mood of peace and humor displayed by the members. Sometimes a whole day would go by without any mention of AMD, as if everyone had forgotten why they were there. Then ninety-one-year-old Bob M., one of the group's veterans, announced that he had finally learned to accept the disease. That's when M. J. said good-bye.

What she didn't understand was that Bob (a decorated Royal Air Force pilot during World War II) was not talking about lying down and dying. He was talking about getting up and living. He finally understood that "acceptance" meant facing the disease as a reality and doing something about it.

In his essay *The Ethics of Belief* (1877), William Clay Clifford wrote, "the method of solution is the other half of the answer."[51] "Why me?"—the despairing question often asked by the newly diagnosed—may be best answered with, "Let's find out." According to Clifford, the process of learning that would follow might actually lead to an *acceptable* answer by which despair would be abolished.

You saw Jim move from depression to acceptance in just a few weeks of low vision rehabilitation. He had enjoyed good eyesight for more than half a lifetime. Then, by courageously facing and learning to deal with his unexpected visual impairment, he gained the strength to go the rest of the way when much of that sight was lost.

The author Dorothy H. Stiefel wrote:

> Now you see, and now you don't. Acknowledge it for what it is: reality. During the first years of "losing" and not fully understanding why, I was the "Angry One." A little later, partially resigned to my "misfortune," I became a bundle of raw frustration: "The Impatient One." One day, after twenty years of experiencing, resigning, and feeling "down" . . . something clicked in my head, and the fight was on! Emotionally battle-scarred, I had definitely become a challenger. The day of reckoning . . . came with a rekindling of a long repressed natural sense of humor.[52]

These people achieved acceptance. In each case, it was a learning process motivated by frustration and fueled by courage. For you, it may come more gently and by a more circuitous route. However it comes, don't be afraid to face the process. That is where you will find the answers that can lead to your own *acceptable* future.

IN A SENTENCE:

> *Through low vision rehabilitation you will learn to maximize your vision and live well with AMD.*

DAY **6**

learning

The TASK of Living with Central Vision Loss

FOCAL POINTS:

- ▶ *You have a disability, but you are not disabled.*
- ▶ *You can find alternative ways to live successfully.*
- ▶ *Your life will be as good as you make it.*

EIGHTY PERCENT of your sensory information is obtained through sight. No wonder it is so traumatic to lose the ability to see well. Normal daily activities like reading the morning paper, pouring coffee, writing checks, watching television, and even getting dressed can become seemingly impossible.

As your vision declines, you have basically two options. You can either allow yourself to become handicapped, or you can find ways to deal with the inevitable problems and live a quality life. That is what Day 6 is about: learning to live well with central vision loss. In this section you will read about:

○ How to recognize signs of depression, and what to do about it
○ Daily living tips from AMD people themselves
○ How to find important support and informational resources

Most people experience an emotional reaction when they are first told they have an incurable retinal disease. Many react in disbelief, or shock, or anger. Others may experience sadness or a sense of loss. And some may think, "Okay, I've got something that's going to make my life more difficult. But it's not going to kill me or cause me physical pain, so I'll just learn to deal with it."

Most people eventually reach that point, but usually not until they have paid an emotional price. You will find, however, that as you begin to adapt, learn about your condition, and share your experiences and feelings with others, your strongest emotions will lessen. Hopefully, those emotions will evolve into a strong determination to not let visual impairment get the best of you. Or worse, beat you. That kind of tenacity is your best defense.

Retinal research is progressing, and breakthroughs are becoming more frequent. A cure for macular disease is going to be found, and there is even hope of someday restoring lost vision. These developments, however, are several years down the road. In the meantime, we may want to maximize our abilities by building a special kind of personal **TASK force**.

The letters **TASK** stand for the four elements of success for a visually-impaired person:

Tenacity: the determination to explore new directions. You can maintain your quality of life if you are persistent in your search for the tools and resources needed to overcome obstacles—even when you are told that nothing can be done.

Adaptability: your willingness to change your way of doing things. You had no choice when it came to losing your eyesight, but you do have choices when it comes to how you are going to live with the difficulties.

Support: from which comes **cope-ability**. Family members, friends, doctors, and organizations can provide the understanding and assistance you need to cope with low vision.

Knowledge: your most effective defense against the onslaught of sight loss. Knowledge puts a face on the enemy and a powerful weapon in your hands

Tenacity

If you are losing your central vision, you are probably reading this book to learn ways to continue leading a full and independent life. That means you are squarely facing the possibility of visual disability and showing the tenacity that is the first element in your personal TASK force.

Some people show their tenacity by working to help others, as many in our Internet community have done. One of those people is Gideon N., who founded a highly successful support organization in Israel. Frances M., at the age of eighty-one, ran a support group in Nevada and appeared on television talk shows to discuss AMD. Dave P. publishes a running account on the MD Support Web site about his life with AMD. People like Linda O., Donna B., and Cliff M. have developed their own Web sites about low vision, responding to e-mail messages from anyone who writes for help. These people have directed their energies toward public service. Others show their tenacity by simply maintaining their way of life as normally as possible: pursuing hobbies, traveling, spoiling grandchildren, volunteering, and even holding down full-time jobs.

All of these men and women know how it feels to be diagnosed with an incurable disease of the retina, and they know how important it is to go on in spite of it. They also know that going on is not only possible, but that the very act of tenacity can sometimes reveal strengths they never knew they had.

The most difficult hurdle for some people is depression. Upon first hearing their diagnosis, many go through a grieving process. This is very common and absolutely normal. It is *not* normal, however, if depression continues for more than a few weeks. That could be serious, and intervention by family members or friends may be necessary.

In their excellent book *Macular Degeneration: The Complete Guide to Saving and Maximizing Your Sight*,[53] Lylas Mogk, MD, an ophthalmologist, and Marja Mogk, PhD, listed the most common symptoms of depression:

○ Frequently feeling apathetic or unmotivated
○ Frequently feeling agitated, empty, or numb
○ Feeling negative about yourself or frequently pessimistic

○ Withdrawing socially
○ Insomnia or hyperinsomnia (that is, sleeping too little or too much)
○ Losing or gaining more than five percent of your body weight in a month
○ Noticeable decrease in energy
○ Unexplained episodes of crying

Everyone has good and bad days. That is to be expected with the ups and downs of a progressive disease like AMD. Sometimes a walk in the park or a phone conversation with a friend is all it takes to feel better. If, however, you have more than your share of the above symptoms and cannot seem to shake them, you may have **clinical depression**. This is a very real medical condition caused by an imbalance of the brain chemicals that control your emotions. It is serious, but it can be alleviated with medication, behavioral adjustment, and/or strong human support. *Do not* try handling depression alone or hiding it from others. That kind of isolation is likely the reason for your depression in the first place. Tell someone. Ask for help.

Depression is a downward spiral that can be turned into an upward spring, but don't try it by yourself.

If you are doing fine, but you notice after a while that people don't always ask how you are doing, or they don't offer as much help as they used to, don't assume that they have stopped caring. It may be simply that they don't know what to do. In that case, lend them this book.

A Message from the AMD Community

DEAR NAN, AMY, CASSIE and whoever else struggles with depression, anxiety, and fear, I have lived with this particular loss for over 30 years. I can remember like yesterday the fear and shock. I wanted more than anything to make it not so. In fact, I spent a significant part of my life trying to hide the truth, and I settled for a lesser self. That lesser self allowed others to believe that I was weird, spacy, rude, and lazy. All this to avoid the truth of low vision. None of us want this to be so. We would do just about anything to make it go away. But the reality is that we have no control over it. Loss is part of life, but we as human beings spend most of our lives trying to avoid it!

Friends, we cannot avoid this, and I believe, in a very real way, that we are blessed because of that. We are depressed and panicked, because we cannot rely totally on ourselves. The beauty of our surroundings begins to fade and eventually disappear. We are stripped of the *do* part of our identity and forced to see, maybe for the first time, what we are really made of. For most of us, that is frightening!

I totally feel the sadness and fear that walk alongside of us every day. I just want to remind us all that it is courage and compassion that bind people together. It is love and acceptance that we will remember. Be gentle with yourselves, and let the honest empathy, without apology, that flows from this group of people be like salve to your hearts, and watch how your world begins to brighten.

Sharon

Another reason might be that since there is no visible sign of your condition, other people are not constantly reminded of your vision, as you are. They may even think you would prefer not to discuss the subject, so if you want to talk about it, bring it up. Just be sure, as with any other topic of conversation, to choose the right time and audience.

You read earlier that tenacity is having the determination to explore new directions. The first steps in that journey may require you to:

Discover and develop your hidden strengths
Maintain a sense of humor and an openness about your feelings
Avoid depression by focusing your energies on positive action and productive activities
Communicate with others

At the same time, you will want to begin building the other three elements of your TASK force: *Adaptability, Support,* and *Knowledge.* These elements can, and should, be initiated simultaneously and as soon as possible.

Until a few years ago, that was very difficult to do, but thousands of people are now finding very timely emotional relief, due to the immediacy of the Internet. In

Week 12 you will read more about how to find information and support online. Through the resources of the World Wide Web, everything you need is within easy reach, either by you, your support group leader, or a family member. You can take comfort in knowing that every question has an answer, and every answer is a strike against the emotional assault of vision loss.

Adaptability

When you were first diagnosed, you were probably told that you might eventually lose some or all of your central vision. You might have thought you would also lose your independence as a result. In all honesty, it is not easy living with central vision loss; but with a few changes in your environment, and with the help of some of those low vision devices Jim wrote about in Day 5, you can continue to live a full and independent life.

Even if your condition progresses to the advanced stage, you will still be able to function with your peripheral vision intact. This means you will still be able to move about unassisted and continue to see the world around you. You will, however, need to make some adaptations.

Because of the loss of your fine detail vision, the first and foremost change may be to *slow down.* It will take a little longer to finish projects and get where you're going, so give yourself the gift of time.

Here are some other tips, shared with you by the people in our AMD community:

If you take walks outdoors, wear a hat with a brim or bill for shade, protect your eyes with 100 percent UV- and near-UV-protective sunglasses.

Wear sensible shoes. You might also consider walking during midday for the best lighting and fewest shadows.

Carry a white cane as a signal to others that you are visually impaired.

In your home, doorways never seem to be wide enough, so when approaching them, use the back of your hand to guide yourself through. This will prevent you from possibly hurting your fingers.

Make sure the task at hand is directly lit.

Avoid scatter rugs, which can cause tripping.

Pick specific places for items, and train family members to put them back. Be organized to keep rooms free of clutter.

Wherever and whenever possible, replace your square tables with tables that have rounded corners.

Keep dining room chairs pushed in.

For everyday meals, consider using disposable plates, cups, and utensils.

Get measuring cups that are of individual sizes, rather than one cup marked with all measurements.

Be sure to keep your dishwasher and cabinets closed.

When moving from one room to another, carry a basket containing necessary items, such as magnifiers and flashlights.

Learn to use your hands and fingers to feel what you used to do by sight.

Drag your laundry in a bag. It's easier and safer than carrying.

Buy clothes that are color-coordinated, but then mix and match.

You can mark the colors on your clothing and shoes with products like "Puff Paint" or "Hi Marks." With such products, you can design certain symbols for certain colors by applying raised dots. They come in a tube and are washable.

Buy same-colored socks that can be matched easily.

Have someone around who will tell you when you have stains on your clothes or other such problems.

You will find many more helpful hints in Month 5.

Low vision devices are also helpful in adapting daily living activities. In Day 5, you read about several low vision devices that are available in stores and on the Internet. You will find contact information for such dealers in Appendix C.

It is important to point out that what works for one person may not work as well for another, and low vision devices can be expensive. For that reason, you will want to try several models before purchasing. A low vision specialist or a rehabilitation specialist can help you, so ask your doctor to recommend one in your area, or contact your state agency for the blind (see Appendix A).

If you are still able to see to read but find normal-sized print to be a problem, you can find large-print materials, which are available from book dealers and on free loan from organizations and libraries (see Appendix D). The *New York Times* offers the news in sixteen-point type, and *Reader's Digest* also offers a large-print version of their publication. Most major publishers create large-print editions when demand justifies the expense. Amazon.com currently lists about thirty thousand such publications now on the market. However, if a title you want is not published in large print, there are companies that, for a fee, will either reprint it for you or download it to your home or library computer so that you can read it using magnification software.

If you own a computer and a scanner, you can enlarge printed material yourself on your monitor screen. A scanner will convert the printed material into a computer file, which you can then open and magnify to any size on your screen. If your computer does not have built-in magnification software, you can purchase brand names such as Jaws, Text Reader, ZoomText, Window Eyes, and Open Book. Information on how to contact dealers may be found in Appendix C. It is important to note again that what works for one person may not work for another, so you might want to take advantage of free trial periods, which are offered by most companies.

If your vision is such that it is difficult to read even large print or magnified text, you might enjoy listening to audiobooks, which are available at no cost from a number of agencies and from the Library of Congress. These books cover a wide selection of subjects, and you will be provided at no charge with a special machine to play them on. Commercial audiobooks sold in stores can be played on any standard cassette tape deck or CD player. Appendix E lists audiobook sources, and Appendix A lists state agencies for the visually impaired, which can assist you further. All of these resources are also freely available and continually updated on the MD Support Web site at www.mdsupport.org.

Adaptability is a very important element of your TASK force. By actively controlling your daily environment, you will be taking a large step toward reducing the challenges of this disease to manageable levels, and the amount of help available to you is constantly growing.

Support

With the rapid growth of the Internet and the formation of support organizations, millions of people around the world are sharing the knowledge and support they need in order to deal with central vision loss. Losing vision is never going to be easy, but it helps a great deal to know that you have lots of company.

Internet e-mail discussion groups, conference rooms, chat rooms, and message boards are excellent ways for you to communicate with others. They can be nearly as immediate as live conversation, and there is always someone who is ready to listen at any time of the day or night. With special computer software, you don't even have to see to type or read. Recent technology will allow you to type a message by speaking into a microphone. A computer can also read aloud the messages you receive. Speech software can be purchased on the Internet or at most computer supply and low vision product stores under brand names like Jaws, Window Eyes, OutSPOKEN, VocalEyes, and Text Reader. You can find names of all such products and their distributors in Appendix C.

At this time, more than twenty-five AMD support organizations can be reached through Web sites, by phone, or through the mail. All of the organizations can be reached through the MD Portal, a page on the MD Support Web site containing direct links to each of them with descriptions of their purposes, activities, organizational structures, and financial condition. Another excellent source of support is the tried and true printed book.

Other books relative to AMD are listed in Month 12. Most can be purchased through your local bookstore or through the Internet.

No matter where you find it, a good support system is vital when living with vision loss. Family members and friends are your most immediate source of support, especially if they are informed about your condition and your needs. Start by sharing this book with them. As discussed in Day 6, some of your best support will come from people who share your condition, or from people who are experienced in assisting the visually impaired. That means finding or starting a group, either on the Internet or in your area, or locating a good rehabilitation counselor. You may feel intimidated by the prospect of joining a group, since it would mean interacting with new people. You will, however, be surprised how easy it is when you have something in common as personal as vision loss. In Month 3, you will find tips on how to find a support group online or in your local area.

Use the same tenacity that has gotten you this far, and try a support group, either on the Internet or in your town. Not only will you be helping yourself, but you will very likely find that you also have something valuable to offer.

Knowledge

The fourth and final element in your TASK force is knowledge. Knowledge yields power. Power, in turn, gives you the confidence to handle whatever comes, secure in knowing that nothing important is slipping by unnoticed. Knowledge ensures you a more balanced partnership with your doctor when discussing and managing your care. You may not carry all you need to know in your head, but you are at least familiar with the important things, and you know where to look for the rest. Knowledge is probably more powerful and effective than the other elements, but it is the easiest to acquire. Until the early 1990s the average person could obtain information about macular disease only from a doctor or a medical library. And then it was widely dispersed and difficult to understand by the layperson. Since then, the Internet has cultivated the sharing of nearly everything written on the subject. Knowledge is literally at everyone's fingertips. Questions are answered almost as soon as they are asked. This immediacy has greatly reduced or eliminated the long period of anxiety and depression that many people formerly endured. There are, of course, inherent pitfalls in the Internet, which is still a giant stew thrown together by millions of cooks with no recipe book. Be street-smart, maintain a bit of healthy cynicism, and always check your sources. That is how to ensure the most accurate information, whether on the Internet, from broadcast and print media, or even from within your social circle.

With so much information available, the temptation is to self-diagnose. That can be dangerous in two ways. First, you will probably think the worst, which can lead to unnecessary distress. Second, you may decide to self-treat, and that can be physically dangerous. Let your doctor do the diagnosis, after which you can follow up with careful research. The best way you can help your doctor help you is to keep yourself informed, ask questions that have been well thought out, and don't hesitate to ask for clarification if necessary.

Tenacity, adaptability, support, and knowledge: these

are the four elements of your personal TASK force. They are strong defenses that, when combined, can help protect you against the physical and emotional assault of vision loss. Living with AMD is no picnic, but many who are traveling this road will tell you that living well is not only possible, but a goal that is well within reach.

Blessings on My Path: Beverly's Story

MACULAR DEGENERATION is something I had heard about all my life, because my mother's family had experienced it before it was better known. Macular degeneration was genetically imposed on me in middle age. I was surprised, because I felt too young to walk down such a path.

For a year or two, waking up each morning was painful. Now, even though my sight is still deteriorating, I cheerfully say good morning. I smile as I swing my legs over the side of the bed. I scramble around for two slippers. I find one of them, and my other foot is searching when I hit my dog's soft muzzle. Jade doesn't complain, but stands and stretches before following me to the kitchen.

Now I face the first challenge of the day: making my morning pot of coffee. I reach and find the coffee canister. I pick up some coffee with the scoop in my right hand. First, I put my left index finger into the scoop. Is the scoop full? If it is, this is my first big success. With my thumb as my guide, I fill the coffee pot.

While the coffee is brewing, I go to the bathroom and wash my hands and face. Brushing my teeth is more tricky than brushing my hair. I've learned to squirt the toothpaste onto my finger and to check the toothbrush to make sure that the bristles are pointed at my teeth. This may seem absurd, but the backside of the toothbrush won't do too much to make my teeth sparkle!

The coffee is brewed! I pour myself a cup. Before pouring, I pause for a second to make sure the cup is right side up.

The coffee was good. Now, I have enough energy to walk down my blind garden path, but first I need to hitch Jade. I will keep walking slowly so that I won't trip or fall.

I do fall purposefully on the green grass, which is comforting. It is soft and sweet. I will sit here and enjoy my sense world. I breathe in the smell of the sweet clover, and I rub a stone and feel its smoothness. Above my head, I hear a robin scolding me, asking me to move away from her nest high up in the branches. My left foot stubs a persistent stone and disturbs it, bringing worms to light.

I move on quietly. I don't want to alarm that robin and her babies. I reach the foot of the path. I stand, looking out across the meadow. I hear in the distance the water from the small stream trickling down from the pine forest. I see the fields dotted with daisies and black-eyed susans. I feel the eyes of the daisies and of the black-eyed susans, and they stare back at me. I am slightly jealous of their seeing eyes!

There was a shower in the night, so it causes the brook to trickle a little more loudly. That water and the early-morning dew make my sneakers squish. I almost enjoy the sound. I watch my footsteps as I move around the wild buttercups. A small gray toad hops across my path and moves away. I take two steps and move homeward. On my left, the toad inspects the bleeding hearts. They politely bow to him. The coral bells sway in the gentle breeze. I can't hear them, but I do hear Jade calling me home. I step through the wooden gate and say good-bye to the flowers, the toad, and the robins.

Back in my kitchen, I pour myself another cup of coffee and count my blessings!

BEVERLY CASTELLINI *wrote this account at age sixty-nine. She and her husband live on the family homestead in the rural area of Hartland, Vermont. In the mid-1960s they built their home on property that her ancestors purchased in 1780. About thirty years later, she was diagnosed with AMD. In spite of, and perhaps because of, her vision impairment, Beverly is compelled to share her literary gifts with the world. She is a lovely example of someone who has succeeded at the TASK of living with central vision loss.*

IN A SENTENCE:

Your TASK force is your best protection. Work diligently on your tenacity, acceptance, support, and knowledge, and you will be an active, able participant in your own health and well-being.

Who Are Those People in the White Coats?

FOCAL POINTS:

▶ *Learn about the types of doctors who are there to help you.*
▶ *Don't let anyone tell you "nothing can be done."*

HAVE YOU ever called your eye care specialist an "optomologist"? Did you think "OD" stood for "Osteopath Doctor?" Did you know that a very small percentage of doctors are actually certified as low vision specialists? If you are a bit confused, you are not alone. The following information should help straighten things out.

Your first eye doctor was probably an **optometrist**. She examined you and fitted you with your spectacles. Optometrists are also licensed in all states to diagnose and treat various eye diseases and to prescribe eye medication. An OD (Doctor of Optometry) degree is required. (That is not to be confused with a DO degree, which is held by a Doctor of Osteopathy.)

If your optometrist sees a problem with your retina, he might refer you to either an ophthalmologist or a retina specialist. An **ophthalmologist** (pronounced "ahf-thal-MOLL-o-jist") is a medical doctor (MD) who is trained in surgery and care of the eye and its related structures. An ophthalmologist is also licensed to prescribe and administer drugs. An MD (Doctor of Medicine) degree is required. A **retina specialist (RS)** is an ophthalmologist who has had additional training in diagnosis and treatment of the retina and vitreous. She would therefore have advanced knowledge about diseases such as AMD.

The medical eye care field is further broken down into specialties in treatment of the vitreous, retina, and macula. Some doctors might specialize in only one area, while others may specialize in two or more.

Once your diagnosis and any possible interventions are determined, you might then be seen by a **low vision specialist (LVS)**. This is an optometrist or ophthalmologist who specializes in the examination, treatment, and management of patients with visual impairment. The LVS may prescribe various treatment options, including low vision devices, and assist you with identifying other resources for vision and lifestyle rehabilitation. As you saw in Day 5 with Jim's story, the services of an LVS do not offer a cure for the causes of low vision, but they do help patients learn how to utilize their remaining vision to its fullest potential. Low vision care does not replace the possible need for other treatments such as laser, medication, and surgery.

If you require additional low vision rehabilitation, you might work with a **certified low vision therapist (CLVT)**. This is a person with a bachelor's degree in a health-related field who has completed further training and passed a national examination. A CLVT is not a doctor, but he works in conjunction with optometrists and ophthalmologists in the implementation of your evaluation and training.

All of these people work in the area of low vision, which is defined as an impairment of sight that cannot be adequately corrected with pharmaceutical or surgical interventions, conventional prescription eyewear, or contact lenses. The patient usually displays loss of visual field, loss of light sensitivity, distortion, loss of color vision, and/or loss of contrast. Low vision varies with each individual and occurs as a result of genetic birth defects, injury, aging, or **complication** from disease.

What to look for in a low vision specialist

There is nothing to prevent a doctor from simply calling himself or herself a "low vision specialist," but there are a few places you can go for crucial information:

○ The Low Vision Section of the American Optometric Association, at (800) 365-2219, will be glad to provide names and numbers of doctors in your area. Membership in this group does not ensure that the doctor is a full-time low vision practitioner. It does, however, indicate that the doctor is particularly interested in this field and is presumably keeping up-to-date with current developments.

○ Your current eye doctor should know of some of the better people locally involved in low vision care. You might also have a local optometric or medical society that may be contacted for such referrals. Just be sure to note that you are looking specifically for low vision help, not just a general eye evaluation.

○ VisionConnection.com is a good Internet resource that will lead you in the right direction. It offers a search feature to locate ophthalmologists and other vision practitioners who are in the field of low vision.

When you do locate one or more low vision doctors, don't hesitate to ask them (call on the phone if you like) about their background in low vision and if they do indeed specialize in this area. Ask them what you can expect from a visit—and don't be shy when it comes to inquiring about fees.

Each examination or evaluation will be a bit different, but in general, at the initial visit the doctor is likely to review your ocular and medical history. It would be helpful if he can obtain copies of recent eye examinations ahead of time. These records can be obtained by writing to your previous examiner and asking that copies be delivered to the requesting doctor's office.

The doctor will want to make sure that your current eyeglasses are up-to-date. She will also want to make sure that any complicating conditions, such as diabetes or glaucoma, are being adequately cared for. If there is some doubt about an accurate diagnosis, special tests may be run, or you may be asked to return to your original doctor for some of these tests. Once it is clear just what your ocular status is, then decisions can be made about how best to proceed.

Every single person can be assisted in some manner, if they wish to be. You should never be told that "nothing can be done." Any time you hear this, disregard it. That is not to say that lost eyesight can be restored, but some level of independence, however small, can still be obtained. Even someone who is totally blind (no light perception at all) can still be told about the free audio-books program provided by the government, and about various reading machines that scan text and convert it to speech. If necessary, patients should be assigned to rehabilitation therapists for assessment of home environments and to assist with low vision devices in the home setting.

In many cases, what the doctor has to offer may not be of interest to the patient, but at least the patient should always have the choice of information. What is important to realize and remember is that there are options available, including magnifiers, large-print objects, and talking devices. If your low vision specialist cannot discuss these with you, it is time to find someone else who can.

Expect to spend some time over several visits with your low vision specialist. It can take time trying to decide what low vision devices, if any, will be suitable for your needs. It is equally important to learn how to use them properly. The best device in the world is useless if you can't operate it correctly. Low vision care is considered part of rehabilitative medicine, and the teaching and learning part is crucial to success. Many patients end up disappointed because they were not instructed properly in the use of the equipment, or they had unrealistic expectations.

It is important to remember that low vision specialists cannot replace lost eyesight in most cases, but they can maximize that which remains. You may be unable to read the large "E" at the top of the eye chart, yet with sufficient magnification you might be able to read large-print books and magazines. This kind of reading, however, can be slow and difficult. It may mean reading only one or two words at a time. It may mean taking a break every few paragraphs. It is not easy, but with effort, many people are able to read their mail and large-print books and magazines (maybe even regular books and magazines), thereby maintaining a fair degree of independence. This is not always possible, but a thorough low vision evaluation should fairly quickly identify what is realistic and what is not. The important thing to remember is that you *can* be helped to some extent or another.

It is also important to realize that only a very small number of patients seen by a low vision specialist are totally blind. In almost all cases, some vision remains. Remember, AMD by itself will not lead to total blindness. Other complicating conditions may possibly lead to such an acute condition (e.g., severe stroke or trauma, or untreated glaucoma), but few AMD patients experience total visual loss.

Tremendous research is ongoing. The coming years will bring major advances in the treatment or prevention of AMD. Whether this comes from genetic work, medical or surgical treatment, or some type of advanced biotechnology, only time will tell. In the meantime, finding a qualified low vision specialist with whom you are comfortable is a step in the right direction and will help improve your quality of life dramatically.[54]

living

Understanding Your Doctor

STORIES ABOUND about overworked and insensitive doctors, and most of those stories portray the patient receiving the short end of the stick. Keeping in mind that the majority of doctors are doing their level best to take care of your needs, here is a scene that takes place all too often:

"I'm Going What?!"

"You're going blind, and there's nothing that can be done," repeated the doctor.

"That's what I thought you said," you reply, blocking his exit.

He tries to step around you. "I'm sorry, but I have a retinal detachment waiting in surgery."

"But I have questions," you plead.

"Please see my nurse," he says. "She has pamphlets."

Holding your ground, you say, "From what I've

read, AMD does not cause blindness, and there are at least three treatments being researched for my type."

"Yes," he says, taking a step back, "that's true."

"So I'm not going blind?"

"That was a figure of speech."

"No, that was more like a compassionless display of ignorance."

"Okay," he sighs, looking at his watch, "you're losing your central vision, but researchers are closing in on treatments and possible cures. Please see my nurse for a pamphlet that will lead you to additional information. May I get to my next appointment now? There are patients here worse off than you."

"There are?" you ask. "You mean I'm still in pretty good shape?"

"You could go years before experiencing significant visual impairment," he admits.

"You know," you say with a tight smile, "the more we talk, the better I feel. Thank you for spending these extra few minutes with me."

"You're welcome," he replies. "Do you mind if I . . . ?"

"Of course not," you say, and he's off to his retinal detachment.

"Good doctor," you muse. "Needs to give himself the gift of time, though." And you set off to reward your little accomplishment with a chocolate malt.

Here are some facts that may help you to understand your doctor's position.

Your doctor usually has more patients than she can handle. The population is growing faster than the number of competent doctors entering the field. The expense of education (including continued training and attendance at conferences) and the high cost of equipment and insurance protection dissuades many young people from going into the eye care profession. Of those that do choose that route, only 5 to 10 percent go on to certification as low vision specialists. The reason? Until recent breakthroughs, there has simply been very little the eye care profession could offer in the way of treatment. No treatment equals a low percentage of repeat business, which equals a low income. Hopefully, with more treatment options now becoming available, the number of low vision specialists will increase.

Your doctor is an eye care professional, not a counselor. He is trained to diagnosis a condition and, if possible, fix it. If you expect more than that, you may be disappointed. You have the right, however, to expect clear communication about your condition and well-informed direction to sources of further information. If your doctor is one of those special people who go beyond your expectations by spending time explaining and offering comforting advice, you are fortunate. If, however, you feel that communication could be better, go to your appointment prepared with a list of questions. Ask that answers be provided either then or later by mail. That is a reasonable request that is fair to both you and the doctor. You will find such a list in Month 2.

If your doctor is with a university hospital, she is expected to take part in research and possibly to teach classes. This is an extra demand of energy and time, which may mean that she will not be available in the clinic five days a week. Your doctor may also practice at more than one clinic, or give presentations at conferences, organizational meetings, and support groups. If the doctor is not in when you call, golf is not likely the reason.

Your doctor is a human being with a desire to help people, but the job can be thankless, especially when dealing with patients with incurable diseases. Why not send a brief note of appreciation after your next appointment? You may never know how much effect that might have, but you can bet you will be remembered the next time you go in.

IN A SENTENCE:

Take time to check the qualifications of your doctor, and don't hesitate to seek a second opinion if you are not satisfied.

FIRST-WEEK MILESTONE

Good for you. You have shown a lot of tenacity and courage by reaching the end of your first week with AMD. This has been the toughest part of your journey, during which you have:

○ SQUARELY FACED AND IDENTIFIED THE TYPES, CAUSES, AND SYMPTOMS OF AMD.

○ DEVELOPED STRATEGIES FOR EDUCATING OTHERS ABOUT YOUR CONDITION.

○ BECOME A MORE EFFECTIVE PARTNER WITH YOUR DOCTOR BY LEARNING THE BASIC ANATOMY OF THE EYE AND HOW TO MONITOR YOUR OWN CONDITION.

○ BECOME ACQUAINTED WITH IMPORTANT EYE HEALTH HABITS FOR SLOWING DOWN THE PROGRESSION OF AMD AND ADDING TO THE QUALITY OF YOUR LIFE.

○ LEARNED HOW YOU CAN MAXIMIZE YOUR VISION AND YOUR DAILY LIFE THROUGH LOW VISION REHABILITATION.

○ LEARNED THE IMPORTANCE OF TENACITY, ADAPTABILITY, SUPPORT, AND KNOWLEDGE IN DEALING WITH VISUAL IMPAIRMENT.

○ BECOME MORE FAMILIAR WITH THE DUTIES OF EYE CARE SPECIALISTS AND THE CHALLENGES THEY FACE.

The War on AMD

FOCAL POINTS:

- *Learn about promising pharmaceutical treatments.*
- *Learn about alternative treatment with nutritional supplements.*

SCIENTISTS HAVE been fighting a fierce war against AMD since it first reared its head as a recognized disease in the late nineteenth century. The enemy has been resistant, but research has yielded some promising treatments since the 1990s.

Battles are being waged on two fronts: **pharmaceutical** and **surgical**. Some of these treatments have been proven, some are in science-based **clinical trials**, and some are considered **alternative,** or **complementary**. All of the leading treatments will be discussed in Weeks 2 and 3, beginning this week with drugs and dietary supplements.

Most drug treatments are for wet AMD. This type accounts for only 10 to 15 percent of cases, but it can cause the quickest and most dramatic vision loss. Researchers, therefore, are most interested in eliminating wet AMD first.

Treatments for dry AMD are also being studied, since it is the precursor of the wet form. Successfully treat dry AMD, and the enemy can be held at bay. Cure it, and the war is over.

Week 2 introduces you to all known pharmaceutical therapies as of this writing. New developments, however, are being announced almost daily. You will want to keep up by periodically consulting reliable sources, such as the organizations listed in Appendix A. Several of them mail out printed newsletters to those who ask, and others provide telephone hotlines. If a support group is nearby, that is another good source of updated information.

Pharmaceutical treatments

PHOTODYNAMIC THERAPY (FOR WET AMD)

Before the year 2000, the only treatment for wet AMD was the use of a "hot" laser to coagulate leaking blood vessels. That procedure is called **laser photocoagulation**. It is still being used in special cases, but is not favored, as it destroys surrounding healthy tissue. **Photodynamic therapy (PDT)**, however, uses low voltage, so very little damage results. This means the procedure can be safely repeated as many times as necessary, but preferably no more often than every six weeks.

The first step in the procedure is *intravenous* injection of the drug *verteporfin*, which is taken up specifically by the abnormal blood vessels in the retina. A low-voltage ("cool") beam of red laser light is then aimed into the eye to activate the drug. The light causes a toxic form of oxygen to be produced from the chemical, which causes the leaking to stop.

PDT is approved in more than fifty countries under a variety of criteria. In the United States it is approved by the **FDA** (Food and Drug Administration) for only the **classic** form of wet AMD. It is sometimes combined with steroids or antiangiogenic drugs for even better results. Side effects are minimal.

ANTIANGIOGENIC DRUGS (FOR WET AMD)

A substance in the body, **vascular endothelial growth factor (VEGF)**, is responsible for the growth of new blood vessels. When the macular cone cells begin to wither, the VEGF goes into action. The vessels do not, however, form properly, so they leak. This causes relatively quick vision loss from scarring of the retina.

The term **antiangiogenic** is a tongue twister that literally means "against blood vessel development." Antiangiogenic drugs prevent the VEGF from forming vessels. Such drugs have been used successfully for treating cancerous tumors, and now they are showing success in the treatment of wet AMD.

An antiangiogenic drug is normally **injected** directly into the eyeball. There is little discomfort from the procedure, and the doctor will carefully watch for any negative side effects, the most common of which are an increase in **intraocular pressure (IOP)** and infection; both can be treated.

Not all antiangiogenic drugs are injected into the eyeball. Some can be **infused** into a vein, and some can be injected into the tissue around the eyeball. The method depends upon the type of drug and, in some cases, doctor preference. This treatment is not a cure, so maintenance injections may need to be administered every few weeks or months.

No matter how painless it is, no one likes the thought of getting a needle in the eye. For this reason and the potential side effects, better methods of drug delivery will likely be available in a few years. Implanted time-release capsules and doctor-administered eyedrops are two methods being considered.

Antiangiogenic drugs were first made available to patients with the introduction of Macugen (pegaptanib sodium) in 2005. A few months later, a second drug, Lucentis (ranibizumab) was shown to not only slow vision loss in an unprecedented 96 percent of the subjects, but to also improve visual acuity in a significant number of those cases.[55] Lucentis was approved by the FDA in June 2006. This was a historic first that promises to be followed by a train of more exciting discoveries in the fight against wet AMD.

SMALL INTERFERENCE RNA (FOR WET AMD)

A different kind of anti-VEGF drug, **small interference RNA (siRNA)**, is showing promise as a different approach to treatment of wet AMD. Instead of blocking the VEGF, as do the antiangiogenics, siRNA actually turns off the gene that creates the VEGF in the first place.[55] The drug is currently under study.

Statins (for dry and wet AMD)

Statins are a type of cholesterol-reducing drug that lower the levels of fats (lipids) in the blood, including cholesterol and triglycerides. Since 2002, research has shown that statins can also be used to slow the progression of AMD. Other studies, however, have suggested that the drugs may do more harm than good.

By lowering cholesterol, statins interfere with the body's response to inflammation. Uncontrolled inflammation has recently been suspected to be a possible cause of AMD, but controlled inflammation is important as a healing mechanism. Inhibiting inflammation without considering the inevitable imbalance in the immune system could contribute to a wide variety of disorders. If you take statin drugs, supplementation with the **enzyme** CoQ10 is one possible solution to the dilemma.

Drug side effects

Drugs can affect different people in different ways. In addition to acting upon a disease, a drug can also cause other conditions called side effects. Some side effects are minor, while others can be dangerous. Some affect a large percentage of people, while others affect only a few. These factors have to be weighed against the effectiveness of the drug to determine if it should be approved for the market. The first phase of a clinical trial (called the "safety and efficacy" phase) is designed to study two things: whether the drug works for a significant majority, and whether it causes any potentially serious side effects.

No approved drug is without side effects. Hopefully, however, they are few and acceptable. One person may develop a temporary headache, while another may experience nausea. At the same time, a third person may have no adverse reactions at all, and that is supposed to be the majority. Before drug treatment is administered, your doctor will advise you of all side effects that showed up in the trials. You will then be asked to sign a consent form to verify that you understand and that you give approval for the treatment. This is called "informed consent," and it is required in every case. Be sure you read thoroughly anything you are given to sign, and don't hesitate to ask questions ahead of time.

You should also be aware of nonophthalmic drugs that can have adverse effects on your eyes. These are drugs you might be taking for other conditions, such as osteoporosis or cardiac problems. You should be aware of side effects from those drugs as well, so read the inserts carefully. Appendix F lists those products that are known to have adverse effect on vision. If you see one that you are taking, discuss your options with both the prescribing physician and your eye doctor.

living

Herbal Remedies and Dietary Supplements: Good Alternatives?

CONVENTIONAL MEDICINE, such as the treatments just described, relies upon the rigors of scientific testing. Another type of treatment, called alternative (or complementary) medicine, relies principally upon empirical evidence and patient testimonials. This is the category that includes herbal medicines and the dietary supplements discussed back in Day 3.

In 1994, Congress exempted dietary supplements from FDA regulation. Such products are now being sold unregulated, with the only legal requirement being that they cannot be promoted as preventions or treatments of disease. This can cause a quandary. When a person is diagnosed with a serious, incurable disease and told there is nothing that can be done, he will probably start looking in every corner for a remedy. That is understandable and forgivable, but it can make him vulnerable to empty promises and dishonest practices.

To make things worse, patients will often not tell their doctors that they are taking unproven remedies. This means the doctor might unknowingly prescribe a medication or supplement that could be harmful or even fatal in combination with it. Reliance upon unproven supplements might also delay a proven treatment that may be more effective. Unproven alternatives may work. After all, every successful treatment begins as an unproven idea. However, if no attempt is made to scientifically establish its safety and efficacy, and money is being made from it, then it will naturally fall under suspicion.

Money is, of course, a stumbling block that can keep a good idea in a locked drawer. How many alternative treatments might be the next medical miracle if the inventor could afford the millions of dollars required for study and approval? This causes a dilemma for a newly diagnosed AMD patient who is not a candidate for any of the few approved treatments.

The best situation for you as the patient would be either (1) the formation of an influential but impartial watchdog agency to police the market, or (2) responsible marketing of safe, well-researched products along with accurate labeling and truth in advertising. Until either or both of those circumstances arise, education is the safest answer. You and your eye care specialist both need to stay aware of the latest research and apply it wisely to your case with careful consideration of the total effect on your body. Your general physician should also be in on significant decisions.

The field has already seen a softening of the boundaries that have traditionally divided conventional and alternative medicine. This can be good, as decisions cannot always be either black or white. Often a doctor will go by the "it can't hurt" philosophy if more traditional methods have failed. This should, however, ultimately be your doctor's decision based upon careful analysis of your case. Your doctor, for instance, may recommend that you take bilberry extract or ginkgo biloba, both of which are herbal remedies purported to be beneficial to the retina. However, they are also blood thinners, so you should avoid them if you have active vessel leakage from wet AMD and you are on anticoagulant medication such as aspirin, clopidogrel (Plavix), dipyridamole, heparin, ticlopidine, or warfarin (Coumadin).

To further illustrate the importance of communication with your doctors, consider the effects of vitamin A, considered to be a powerful antioxidant. Your eye care specialist may recommend it as part of the AREDS-recommended formula for retinal health. Your general practitioner, however, may know that you have a liver condition that could be worsened by vitamin A and knows you should not take it.

These are good examples of why, if you decide to try alternative medicine on your own, you need to let all of your doctors know. You may feel awkward about sharing the information, especially if it meets with disapproval, but keeping your doctors in the loop is your best course of action. You will be respected for doing so if you can show that you have carefully researched the therapy. Informing your doctors is not only wise for your health, but it will also provide an additional record by which the effectiveness of the treatment may be measured.

IN A SENTENCE:

*Proven pharmaceutical treatments and some
alternative drug therapies are making strides in the
fight against AMD. Educating yourself about all
options and working as a partner with your doctors
will give you the best advantage.*

Surgical Treatments and Interventions

FOCAL POINTS:

▸ *Learn about promising surgical procedures.*
▸ *Learn about alternative interventional therapies.*

THE SURGICAL treatments and interventions discussed here are for treatment of wet or dry AMD. All are experimental at this time, but scientifically controlled trials are showing promise.

Macular translocation (for wet AMD)

Simply put, **macular translocation** is an experimental surgical procedure that involves detachment of the retina and relocation of it to a healthier spot in the eye.

Researchers at Duke Eye Center in Durham, North Carolina, have been reporting success since 2003 with a refinement of macular translocation.[57] Called "macular translocation surgery with 360-degree peripheral retinectomy" (MT360), it is a two-stage procedure. The first stage involves rotating the retina to move the macula away from the abnormally growing blood vessels. The second stage corrects the resulting tilted visual field by rotating the eye itself.

According to Duke researchers, success is being shown even in people who have experienced scarring and further vision loss after treatment by other means.

Retinal cell transplantation (for restoring vision loss)

While science is a long way from transplanting an entire eyeball, methods of retinal transplantation are being developed for restoring sight to the blind. In August 2004, researchers at the University of Louisville reported that they had successfully and without complications performed a fetal-cell transplant on a sixty-four-year-old woman with retinitis pigmentosa (a disease of the rod cells leading to peripheral vision loss).[58] The subject's visual acuity in the treated eye was 20/800 before surgery. After two years, she could read large-print materials with the surgically corrected eye.

The researchers accomplished this feat by transplanting both the photoreceptor cells and the underlying RPE cells in tandem. This maintained the nourishment of the rods and cones as they gradually took the place of the old cells. The trials continue under FDA supervision and with the approval of the University of Louisville Human Studies Committee.

Remember that retinal cell transplantation is not appropriate for people who still have usable vision. The research will, however, hopefully lead to more refined restoration of macular function in AMD patients.

Drusen lasering (for dry AMD)

Ophthalmologists have taken an interest in using the low-intensity lasers to destroy drusen. The hope is that ridding the retina of these deposits may slow the development of AMD, or even stop the progression from the dry form to the wet form.

A two-year study in 1999 showed promising results,[59] but a follow-up study in 2002 found that laser treatment showed no beneficial effect in preventing choroidal neovascularization (CNV), and may actually promote CNV events and vision loss, at least in the short term.[60] Patients who have drusen in both eyes, with no occurrences of CNV, may or may not benefit from drusen lasering. Research in this field is ongoing.

Vitrectomy (for surgery on the retina)

At this point, it is important that you understand an important part of the procedure for operating on the retina. In order to access the retina, the vitreous gel must be removed and then replaced after surgery. The removal procedure is called a **vitrectomy**.

The operation is usually performed on an outpatient basis. Either silicon oil or a gas bubble is injected into the eye to hold the retina in place until the body replaces the vitreous naturally. Until that happens, it is frequently necessary for the patient to remain in a facedown position.

Vision improvement could take several weeks to a few months. It is important not to be alarmed by blurry vision. The gas bubble will hinder normal focusing until it dissolves of its own accord within a few weeks. The majority of people return to their work and normal lives in one to four weeks following the operation.

living

Alternative Medicine: Interventional Treatment

IN WEEK 2 you read about one type of alternative, or complementary, medicine: herbal remedies and dietary supplements. The second category is defined as interventional treatments that have not been proven by the experimental method. Such procedures have not been sanctioned by the FDA. They are, therefore, not covered by Medicare or other insurance providers.

The most well-known alternative interventional treatments include acupuncture, microcurrent stimulation, chelation therapy, and homeopathy. Each of them will be described here so that you will be able to make informed decisions as to whether a particular procedure might be beneficial to you. Remember, it is very important that you inform your diagnosing doctor about any treatment you undergo outside of his or her purview.

Acupuncture

The original Taoist thinking behind acupuncture is that energy (called Qi, pronounced "chee") is constantly flowing through the body along pathways called "meridians." When the meridians are disturbed in any way, illness can result. Those places where the meridians are close to the surface of the skin are called acupuncture points. That is where very fine needles are inserted to help restore the circulation of Qi, thus restoring a balance between the forces of "Yin" and "Yang" (the two opposing universal forces that comprise Qi).

Researchers have yet to explain acupuncture on a scientific basis, but more than five thousand years of empirical evidence indicates that it works for some conditions, including (perhaps indirectly) retinal disease. Some possibilities are that the treatment raises immunity levels, increases secretion of endorphins, increases levels of serotonin and other neurotransmitters, improves circulation, and controls the "gates" (nerve cells and fibers) that determine levels of pain and paralysis. Acupuncture treatment might also include electrical stimulation, heat from "moxibustion" of certain herbs, or massage therapy (called "acupressure"). However, research has yet to demonstrate improvement in the retinas of AMD patients treated with acupuncture. For more information about this treatment, visit www.acupuncture.com.

One type of acupuncture, called "microacupuncture," is being offered by a few practitioners specifically for people with retinal disease. It involves forty-eight or so "newly discovered" acupuncture points in the hands, feet, and forehead. Again, no scientific basis is offered for the alleged improvements in vision.

Microcurrent stimulation

Microcurrent stimulation (MCS) is a form of electrical acupuncture involving small currents of electricity applied at points around the eyes and elsewhere on the body. Expectations are that the stimulation will boost the cells' ability to rid themselves of waste products and raise the levels of nourishment and oxygenation by increasing blood flow. After approximately seven office visits during the first two weeks of treatment, the patient continues self-treatment using a portable microcurrent machine purchased for home use. The machine is called TENS (Transcutaneous Electrical Nerve Stimulation), and it is in common use in the medical field for treatment of pain. Due to the absence of safety trials, however, the FDA has warned against use of the TENS device to treat retinal disease. In spite of these warnings, practitioners continue to promote MCS as a safe and effective method for treating macular degeneration and other retinopathies. Be aware that any use of an unapproved device is deemed by the FDA as "off-label" and may not be advertised as an approved therapy for AMD. If an alternative device is used off-label, you must be warned by the practitioner that it has not received FDA approval for efficacy and safety.

One company has been working with the FDA to allow legal marketing of an evolved version of the TENS machine. The TheraMac, developed by Acuity Medical, has shown early success for use in what the developer calls biocurrent therapy (to differentiate it from MCS); and FDA open-label and feasibility studies have found the device to be safe and effective. Premarket approval studies are ongoing.

Chelation therapy

Chelation therapy is an intravenous therapy using the synthetic amino acid EDTA (ethylene diamine tetra-acetic acid), which has the ability to bond with atoms of calcium, lead, cadmium, mercury, and some of the trace minerals. These minerals, combined with the EDTA, are eliminated from the body through the kidneys into the urine.

Chelation therapy is used for patients with heavy-metal poisoning, poor circulation due to arteriosclerosis, and related conditions. Arteriosclerosis and the formation of free radicals are thought to contribute to AMD, and chelation therapy has been documented to improve both conditions. More information about chelation therapy may be obtained by contacting the American College for Advancement of Medicine at (949) 583-7666 or by visiting www.acam.org.

Rheopheresis

Rheopheresis is a process much like blood donation, except that rheopheresis removes potentially toxic high molecular weight **proteins** from the blood. Practitioners think these proteins may hinder the delivery of nutrition to the retina. Through rheopheresis, it is thought that blood quality is restored, thus improving its availability to the retina.

Patients recline in a chair for the procedure. An IV line is established in both forearms, and blood is circulated through the filtering equipment. The procedure has been shown to be safe, with the most common side effects being fatigue and dizziness.

Rheopheresis is available in Canada, but the cost per treatment is high for noncitizens. It is not yet approved for use in the United States, so it is not covered by Medicare or other insurance providers.

Homeopathy

Homeopathy is the practice of encouraging your body to heal itself through its own natural defenses (such as your immune system). This is done by ingesting remedies that contain minute doses of the agent thought to cause your illness. Low- to medium-potency remedies may be found in health food stores for acute diseases such as colds and flu, and you may see advertisements for higher-potency homeopathic remedies by prescription for AMD. Be aware, however, that most practitioners will tell you that no homeopathy has been shown to be effective for this condition.

IN A SENTENCE:

> *You will hear about a good number of surgeries and other interventions for treating AMD. It is up to you and your doctors to decide what is best for you.*

More Answers to Important Questions

FOCAL POINT:

▶ *Miscellaneous questions that need answering*

BY THIS time, you may feel as if you've spent a week on a speeding train. This might be a good time to stop for a breather and catch up on anything that might have been passed by. Today will be spent answering remaining important questions that are often asked by newly diagnosed patients.

How long will I keep my eyesight?

Each person progresses at their own rate, so this is a difficult question to answer. Dry AMD progresses very slowly, which means you could retain usable vision for years. However, if the disease advances to the severe wet form, only immediate treatment will keep you from losing vision rapidly (see Day 5).

Remember, you can also be proactive in keeping your eyesight for as long as possible. Proper nutrition, eye protection, and health habits are effective in maintaining your optimum retinal condition (see Day 4).

Should I get a cane or a guide animal?

A cane might be helpful, but guide animals are a precious commodity reserved for the most severely visually impaired. The fortunate fact is that AMD people simply don't need them, even if there were plenty to go around and qualifications allowed ownership.

Barring secondary complications, you will never need a guide animal. Cane training, however, would give you an extra advantage, especially in unfamiliar public places. Training is important for correct technique and safety, so be sure to seek professional guidance if you choose to go that route. You can find orientation and mobility (O and M) trainers at low vision rehabilitation centers (see Appendix A), or ask your doctor for a referral.

Should I learn Braille?

If you have the time and persistence it takes to learn, the answer is a definitive "yes." If your condition progresses to total central vision loss, you will have difficulty reading normal print. Knowing how to read and write in Braille would be a real plus, and a good time to begin learning is while you still have vision.

For information about Braille training, contact the

Hadley School for the Blind in Winnetka, Illinois (Telephone: (800) 323-4238; Web site: www.hadley-school.org). The school offers both live and online courses.

Will cataract surgery make my AMD worse?

In the hands of an experienced surgeon, cataract surgery is usually safe for patients with retinal **dystrophy,** but it can exacerbate wet AMD. Most doctors will recommend that AMD patients wait until the cataracts cause serious vision loss before having the procedure done.

Will cataract surgery improve my eyesight?

Yes, it can help you to see better. Cataract surgery involves removing the cloudy lens of your eye. It is replaced with a new one that is clear of defects and not yellowed from natural aging. This not only helps you to see better, but it also allows the doctor to examine your retina more easily.

Where can I get help paying for my eye care?

At one time or another, everyone needs help. With the high cost of medical care and prescriptions, it is good to know that there is assistance for those who qualify. A reasonable first step is to inquire about assistance from a social worker at a local hospital or community agency. Your doctor should be able to guide you to these resources. Next, you can try state agencies, which are listed in Appendix A.

If you need assistance with paying for drug therapy, contact the pharmaceutical company that makes the drug. Most of them have plans designed to help those who qualify based on income and other measurements of need.

Finally, try contacting the organizations listed in Appendix B. Each has its own requirements and limitations, but you just might be able to make use of such a service. A helpful Web site is NeedyMeds.com, which lists complete information about such programs. If you need help with applying, try going to www.themedicineprogram.com. For a nominal fee, this nonprofit service will assist you.

Is air travel bad for my eyes?

There is no evidence that air travel in a pressurized cabin will harm your retinas under normal circumstances. Your blood pressure, however, might increase if you are stressed by flying. This could be detrimental for people with wet AMD. In addition, patients who have undergone recent vitrectomy surgery should avoid air travel.

Are there drugs that might make my vision worse?

Yes. Drugs that are known to cause potential harm in AMD patients are listed in Appendix F. Be sure your doctor is aware of any and all drugs you take.

Is it possible to transplant an eyeball?

This question arises frequently. Such an operation would be very complex, and it is not possible with today's technology. The main problem is the optic nerve, which contains more than a million connections between the retinal ganglia and the brain. Transplantation of individual parts of the eyeball, however, is not only possible, it is also being done successfully in many cases.

Many of your most pressing questions should have been answered by this time, or you should at least know where to look for further information. So now that you have had this short breather, it's time to move on. There is a lot more ahead.

FIRST-MONTH MILESTONE

Congratulations on reaching the end of your first month. During these past weeks, you have made further strides toward dealing with AMD by learning about:

- O PHARMACEUTICAL TREATMENTS THAT ARE BEING DEVELOPED THROUGH SCIENTIFIC RESEARCH

- O THE POTENTIAL OF HARM TO YOUR EYESIGHT FROM SOME DRUGS

- O SURGICAL PROCEDURES AND IN-TERVENTIONS BEING TESTED

- O ALTERNATIVE TREATMENTS AND THEIR PLACE IN THE FIELD OF EYE CARE

Questions to Ask Your Doctor

FOCAL POINTS:

- ▸ *Communicating efficiently with your doctor*
- ▸ *The risk factors for developing AMD*

A COMMON problem that you might have encountered during these past few months is what to ask your doctor. Your diagnosis probably took you by surprise, and you may have never even heard of AMD before.

To compound the issue, many doctors do not have the time to educate you about all of the aspects of your condition. Your responsibility, therefore, is to learn as much as possible so that you can ask questions about your particular case.

Do not expect your doctor to provide a great deal of emotional support. Instead, expect a courteous professional who knows how to take care of your physical needs. You also have the right to expect someone who is familiar enough with the resources to direct you to other information you might need.

Your doctor is busy. He cannot spend an inordinate amount of time with you, but he will take the time to answer your questions if you are well prepared and concise. That is the purpose of Month 2: to provide you with a basic script. Take this book and a pen with you to your next appointment. The script below will help you to get the answers you need. Write in the doctor's answers or ask that someone write them in for you so that you can study them later in your own good time. If you need help understanding the doctor's responses you may consult the index and the glossary of this book.

You may not like some of the answers, but remain positive. You have probably lived long enough to realize that most things will never be as good as you hope, but neither will they be as bad you think.

Dear Doctor

Please take a few minutes to answer these questions. This will save valuable time during my appointment and allow me to better understand my condition.

1. WHAT STAGE OF AMD AM I IN?
   Left eye (OS):
   [ ] early dry
   [ ] intermediate dry
   [ ] advanced dry
   [ ] subfoveal wet

[ ] juxtafoveal wet
[ ] extrafoveal wet

Right eye (OD):
[ ] early dry
[ ] intermediate dry
[ ] advanced dry
[ ] subfoveal wet
[ ] juxtafoveal wet
[ ] extrafoveal wet

2. **IF I HAVE SUBFOVEAL WET AMD, WHICH SUBTYPE DO I HAVE?**
Left eye (OS):
[ ] predominantly classic
[ ] occult
[ ] minimally classic

Right eye (OD):
[ ] predominantly classic
[ ] occult
[ ] minimally classic

3. **WHAT TESTS DID YOU USE TO CONFIRM MY DIAGNOSIS?**
[ ] acuity exam (Snellen or other chart)
[ ] internal ocular examination
[ ] fluorescein angiogram
[ ] indocyanine green angiogram
[ ] ocular coherence tomography (OCT)
[ ] scanning laser ophthalmoscopy
[ ] other_____

4. **WHAT IS MY ACUITY?**
Uncorrected:
Left (OS): _____ Right (OD): _____ Both (OU): _____

Corrected:
Left (OS): _____ Right (OD): _____ Both (OU): _____

5. **WHAT ARE MY TREATMENT OPTIONS?**
[ ] laser photocoagulation
[ ] photodynamic therapy with Visudyne
[ ] photodynamic therapy with Visudyne + steroid
[ ] steroid only
[ ] antiangiogenic (VEGF blocker) drug therapy
(identify:)_____
[ ] combination drug therapy
(identify:)_____
[ ] none
[ ] other_____

6. **WHAT NUTRITIONAL SUPPLEMENTS DO YOU RECOMMEND?**
[ ] none
[ ] AREDS formula only
[ ] multisupplement containing AREDS formula
[ ] multisupplement only
[ ] lutein (dosage: _____)
[ ] zeaxanthin (dosage: _____)
[ ] statins (dosage: _____)
[ ] Omega-3 (dosage: _____)

[ ] CoQ10 (dosage: _____)
[ ] other:
_____

_____

7. **WHERE CAN I GO LOCALLY TO RECEIVE ASSISTANCE WITH LOW VISION DEVICES AND OTHER LOW REHABILITATION TRAINING?**

_____

_____

8. **DO YOU HAVE INFORMATIONAL HANDOUTS THAT I CAN TAKE HOME WITH ME, SUCH AS THE SMARTSIGHT HANDOUT FROM THE AMERICAN ACADEMY OF OPHTHALMOLOGY?**

_____

_____

9. **HOW OFTEN SHOULD I BE EVALUATED?**

_____

_____

This information from your doctor will give you an excellent start toward understanding and coping with your condition.

Two questions your doctor cannot answer

Some questions simply do not have answers, so you can avoid frustrating both you and your doctor by not asking them. They are:

1. WILL I LOSE ALL OF MY CENTRAL VISION?

Cells degenerate at different rates of speed in different people. Macular degeneration is a progressive disease, but stabilization for months or years can drastically slow down its progression. Therefore, complete loss of central vision could take anywhere from weeks (in some wet macular degeneration cases with no treatment) to years, or degeneration may never reach its full potential if your life span is shorter than the course of the disease.

2. WHEN ARE THEY GOING TO FIND A CURE?

A great deal of research is going on in many areas, giving reason to hope for a cure within the next decade. Any more accurate prediction than that is purely guesswork. The best you can do right now is to practice good nutritional habits, avoid pollution and smoking, protect your eyes from the sun, and stay informed about possible treatments. When the cure does come, you will have done the best you can to take advantage of it.

Will my children and grandchildren develop AMD?

This question has an answer. It is a bit involved, however, so do not expect your doctor to have time to discuss it at length. This section will introduce you to current thinking about the risk factors for developing AMD.

In its "Global Report 2005," the AMD Alliance International divides the risk factors into two categories: "avoidable" and "unavoidable."[61] Avoidable risk factors are those aspects of your life you can control. These, as discussed in Day 4, are diet, health practices, and environment.

Unavoidable risk factors are genetics, aging, gender, ocular abnormalities, ethnicity, and iris color.

GENETIC INHERITANCE OF AMD

Inheritance is an unavoidable risk factor that plays a major role in the development of AMD. This will give you a general introduction to a complicated subject.

For a long time, studies have suggested that genetic predisposition is one of the risk factors for AMD. Finally, between the years 2000 and 2005, two gene discoveries have supported that research.

Four separate 2005 studies identified a gene named "complement factor H" (CFH).[62, 63, 64, 65, 66] All four studies found that this protein limits the immune response and inflammation, but a defect in the gene can cause inflammation to go out of control. The presence of the defective gene raises the risk of AMD two to seven times, with the greatest risk occurring in people with both genes of the pair defective.

There has also been a good deal of excitement about the possible connection between the blood level of C-reactive protein (CRP) and AMD. CRP is responsible for the healing benefit of inflammation that occurs when a part of the body is in trouble. If, however, the level of the protein is elevated, it can cause damage. In a 2004 study, researchers found significantly higher C-reactive protein levels in patients with AMD. Those subjects had a 65 percent higher risk of developing AMD than those with the lowest CRP levels.

These discoveries indicate that anti-inflammatory agents such as aspirin and statin drugs might help to prevent AMD. More important, identification of high levels of CFH and CRP in the body may serve as a **marker** for potential development of the disease. If, as scientists are beginning to discover, AMD is related to the immune system, researchers may be able to develop drugs that focus on that particular response as a partial cure for the disease. More research is needed, and other causal factors, such as environment and nutrition, also need to be considered.

AMD is divided into "early onset" and "age-related." The early onset forms (e.g., Stargardt's disease, Best disease, Sorsby's macular dystrophy) are certainly inherited. Whether or not AMD is inherited, however, is still open to question. Genetic **mutations** are now thought to cause up to half of the cases, but environmental factors and poor health habits are also highly suspect.

In some families, AMD is thought to be an **autosomal dominant** disease. This is a rare situation that means you might have one altered (mutated) gene paired with one normal gene lying on one of twenty-two pairs of autosomal **chromosomes.** You would, therefore, have a 50 percent chance of passing along the altered gene (i.e., the disease) to each of your children.

A person, however, could have the altered gene but not develop the disease. The gene is then said to have **reduced penetrance**, meaning it has somehow been rendered harmless. A person could also have the altered gene and not develop symptoms. This gene has **variable expressivity**, with its effect differing in severity from one affected family member to the next.

Age of onset can also differ among affected people. Some may show symptoms in their thirties, while others might not become **symptomatic** until much later in life. In the latter case, a person could actually have the altered gene but not live long enough to develop the disease. If a child of that person then develops AMD, it would seem (inaccurately) that the disease had skipped a generation.[67]

So will your children or grandchildren become visually impaired from AMD? If you have the rare autosomal dominant form, the chance of passing along the disease is 50 percent. If your condition is not genetic, the question is difficult to answer. If, however, your family has a history of AMD, other influences may be at play, such as environment, dietary habits, and secondary physiological problems. In such cases, the odds of developing the disease can be significantly lowered by attention to recommended eye health practices and frequent retina exams. Add to that the speed with which treatments and potential cures are developing, and it may just be a moot question. That is the hope for your children, and it is a near certainty for the generations to come.

Information on the remaining five risk factors is summarized here from the abovementioned AMD Alliance International report:

Aging
AMD is clearly linked to aging. Prevalence increases from 12.2 percent in people aged 55–64 years to 18.3 percent in those aged 65–74 years and 29.7 percent in people aged over 74. It is important to note that not all of these will be cases of advanced AMD resulting in vision loss. In fact, the figure for those with advanced AMD above the age of 75 is 7.8 percent.[68]

Gender
You may hear that more women than men develop AMD. However, no strong evidence backs this up.[69] For

that matter, a Japanese study has found the prevalence to be higher in men.[70]

Ocular abnormalities

AMD has been linked to **hyperopia** (farsightedness) and a lower cup/disc ratio.[71] (The **cup/disc ratio** is the area of the level part of the optic disc divided by the area of the deep part, or cup, of the optic disc.) Whether or not these conditions are strong predictors of AMD is yet to be determined.

Ethnicity and iris color

To what extent ethnic groups differ in their susceptibility to AMD is difficult to establish. Caucasians, however, are generally considered more likely than others to develop and progress to the advanced stages of the disease.[72] In addition, people with blue or hazel eye color appear to have a higher risk.[73]

IN A SENTENCE:

Knowing what questions to ask and what answers to expect will not only create a good rapport with your health care provider, it will benefit your ongoing health and well-being.

Now What?

FOCAL POINTS:

- *You don't have to deal with this by yourself.*
- *You can be as successful as you want to be.*

Join a support group

Once people who care about you understand your condition, they will want to do everything they can to help. Family members are your most immediate support base. Friends and acquaintances will empathize with you and periodically ask how you are doing. This social circle has served you well for most of your life. Now, however, your circle will need to include people who can offer support from their own experience with AMD.

At least one study has indicated that your

health may improve as a result of access to information and by participating in a support group with others who share your condition. Speculation is that when you become actively involved in your own care, your health will benefit. AMD support group leaders consistently report that the length of time between diagnosis and acceptance is greatly diminished in people who interact with others.

FROM A HAPPY SUPPORT GROUP MEMBER

My e-mail support group is truly an amazing collection of people. When one of us asks the group about a medical condition there are almost always people on hand who know something about it. And if the members don't know it, our leader will probably be able to point us in the right direction.

This is a very powerful thing. The collective wisdom of this group is far, far more than the individual knowledge or wisdom of any one of us. It assures me a better level of treatment. When I go to my doctor armed with information, I am more engaged, able to listen more intelligently to what he says, and able to ask intelligent questions.

My support group provides me with knowledge, which enables me to be a better patient and to have a real dialogue with my doctor. As we tell new members, "The more you know, the more the doctor is likely to talk. Ask us questions. We are here. There is always someone on duty!"

—D. RUCHMAN

If you would like to locate a low vision support group, here are a few suggestions:

Ask your doctor.

Call local retirement centers, churches, or libraries. You may find that one of them is an affiliate of MD Support's National Low Vision Support Group.

Contact your state's low vision rehabilitation agency. (See Appendix A for contact information.)

If you are a veteran, contact the ophthalmology department of a Veterans Administration hospital.

Go to Vision Connection (www.visionconnection.org) on the Internet.

Join the world's largest and longest-running e-mail discussion group about AMD, MD Support, at www.mdsupport.org.

If you are unable to connect with a support group through one of these means, you can form your own group in your home with just a few people and a plate of refreshments. Post a sign in your local community center, at your church, the local Y, your library, or in your newspaper. Ask your eye doctor to spread the word and/or post a sign in her office. This book may be used as a good discussion starter and as a resource for ideas and programs.

Ways your family and friends can help

A support group is an excellent source of understanding and information, but it can never replace caring family members and friends. Lifelong relationships can provide you with the important sense of security and strong emotional foundation that will help you deal with AMD. A solitary disease such as this can cut you off from that vital lifeline, so you will want to strengthen the connection by actively keeping your family and friends involved. Here are some ways to do that:

Ask them to help you with transportation to the doctor, grocery store, etc. Be sure not to wear out anyone in particular. Spread it around, and offer to pay for the gas, too.

Tell them you would like to be invited to social functions, even if you don't always accept their invitations.

Send cards on special occasions, and include a note about how you are doing. Keep it positive and upbeat.

Call for no reason other than to keep in touch.

Invite them over for a simple dinner and conversation.

Tell them frequently how important they are to you— not just in dealing with AMD, but in every other way as well.

Thank them for their efforts in keeping you abreast of the latest research developments, even if you have already heard about it through that excellent support group you belong to.

Ask them to help you with duties around the house that are difficult for you. Then repay them with a big piece of pie or a hug—either one is good.

Ways to keep busy

You won't always be able to depend upon others for company. Those days can be the most difficult, because you will be alone with your thoughts. To avoid slipping

> ## A Message from the AMD Community:
> ## What We Need Most
>
> ### BY SEYMOUR ROB ROBINS
>
> TOO MANY of us lose this battle by default. We become aware that certain things in our lives have been brusquely taken away. No point in going to museums with our friends, but in giving up the museum trips we also give up our friends. Cooking a great meal for guests doesn't happen, because shopping means having to ask someone to take us. Divesting ourselves of these lifelong activities is bad enough, but usually our relationships are where the real loss occurs.
>
> What we need most is people! I don't necessarily mean helpers and caregivers, though they are comforting and necessary at times. We need people for an active and continuing contact with life. Friends must be actively pursued.
>
> Perhaps this is the time we have always wished for. Time for lectures or concerts, or readings or discussions. We must seek an ongoing traffic with people, and it is up to us to initiate and pursue that activity as a means of securing and continuing our own personalities and lives.

into negativism and even depression, you need to keep your time filled with purposeful activities that will get you out of bed in the morning.

To help you get started, the people of the AMD

Internet Community have put together a checklist of ideas that have worked for them. Here they are, in no particular order, straight from men and women who have found ways to remain vital and productive in spite of their impaired vision.

Purchase descriptive videos, which include narration to accompany the movies. For information, contact Descriptive Video Service in Boston at (800) 333-1203.

Listen to broadcasts of magazines and newspapers from In Touch, a subsidiary of the Jewish Guild for the Blind. Membership is free for Medicaid recipients. For more information, call (800) 456-3166 or go to www.intouchnetworks.org.

Listen to National Public Radio. You can learn about it at www.npr.org.

Listen to books and periodicals on tape. See Appendix E for a listing of distributors.

While listening to those tapes, do something physical to stay in shape. Floor exercises, weight lifting, stretching, or yoga will improve your body while you entertain your mind.

Enroll in low vision rehabilitation training for help in maximizing your capabilities. Medicare will usually pay for this. For information, contact your state's agency for the blind, which you can find listed in Appendix A.

Attend concerts, lectures, book readings, and other events. Your church, parks department, or senior citizens group may offer group outings to places such as these.

Start a garden (indoors or out).

Take a class in water aerobics, meditation, or body conditioning.

Become active in your church or local clubs and organizations.

Tape-record your life history for your children and grandchildren.

Take classes in Braille. It will open up a whole new world to you.

Ride a tandem bike or go canoeing with your spouse or a friend.

Learn to play a musical instrument by ear.

Cook and bake. Begin with something simple and familiar until you gain confidence. It may take longer than it used to, so be patient, enjoy the moment, and be ready to forgive yourself for little mistakes.

Go for walks with a pet.

Do large-print jigsaw puzzles, word search puzzles, and crosswords. Reliable evidence shows that such activities also help to ward off dementia in later years. The AARP has a Web site with several free games you can play, including crosswords and jigsaw puzzles, and they change often. The *New York Times* prints all of their crossword puzzles in large-print books, which can be purchased from major booksellers or online at Amazon.com. You can also contact other companies, such as the Senior Store, that deal in large-print materials. These three resources and many more are listed in Appendix C.

learning from living

Driving and AMD

FOCAL POINTS:

‣ *One of the most difficult changes in your life may be giving up driving.*
‣ *You have safer and more economical alternatives to personal transportation.*

CONSIDER THESE facts:

42,636 people were killed in 2004 as a result of traffic crashes.[74]
2,959,295 motor vehicle occupants were injured in crashes during 2001.[75]

If you are an average driver of a midsize automobile, you spend more than six thousand dollars a year (not counting purchase price and finance charges) for the "privilege" of driving.[76]

Think about it: If you have to give up driving, visual impairment may save your life or limbs. It will definitely save you money. (To be fair, you should also know that 170,272 pedestrians were injured in 2001 by motor vehicles,[77] so be extra careful crossing those streets.)

With all of these negatives involving motor vehicles, why on earth would a person want to drive one? When should you stop driving? What does the law have to say about it? What alternatives do you have? Since AMD will obviously affect your ability to drive, you need to think about these questions. These are the topics of discussion this month.

Why drive?

The reasons most mature drivers give for driving (in order of importance) are:

Convenience
Independence
Comfort
Privacy
Pride of ownership

These are all good rationales. Your entire adult life has been spent slipping into the driver's seat whenever the mood or necessity has arisen. Traveling anywhere at any time and staying as long as you liked. Transporting entire trunkloads of Christmas presents at once. Listening to whatever you like on the radio, and even singing along at the top of your voice.

Whether you favor hot rods or minivans, dragster pipes

or a standard muffler, cherry red or clover green, that car is an extension of *you*. You even *named* the thing. "What will life be worth without Betsy?!" you cry.

Get a grip. It's only a car.

That may be a bit blunt, but when you stack your rationales against killing or injuring yourself or someone else, it may be time to put Betsy up for adoption. You gave up cigarettes and high-fat desserts, didn't you? Well, this will be just as difficult but at least as good for you. And you may be surprised at how well you can live without her.

When is it time to give up the keys?

You are the best judge of when driving is no longer safe. Don't wait until you have an accident. Here are some signals that might mean driving is not for you:

You are nervous behind the wheel.

You feel that you react too slowly due to your vision.

You have trouble reading street signs.

You have had a near mishap because you didn't see a pedestrian, an object, or another vehicle.

You get lost easily.

Oncoming lights temporarily blind you.

The sun hurts your eyes, but dark lenses make it difficult to see.

You find it abnormally difficult to see at dusk or dawn.

Your color perception is diminished.

People whom you trust recommend it. (Sometimes they notice things you don't.)

Some people wait one accident too long to admit that they should quit driving. Here is a message from someone it happened to.

The Day I Quit Driving

Condensed from an essay by Joel Deutsch

The phone on the night stand rang, shattering my last dream of the morning.

"Hullo," I mumbled. It was the woman from the Substitute Unit of the L.A. Unified School District. I was to fill in for an English teacher at a middle school halfway downtown.

I didn't know how much more substitute teaching I could take. By this time, my eyesight was severely compromised. And this trip would be straight into the sun. Another harrowing commute. I had the Beverly Boulevard route to the school pretty much hammered from long experience. Whether I could see the traffic lights at first glance or not, I knew which cross streets had them, and I'd become pretty good at telling the color of a light by watching traffic.

I made it through all the major intersections, talking myself down the road. Finally, I took a left into the street and began to peer along the curb for a parking space. I couldn't have been going 10 mph.

Suddenly, I heard the sickening thud of my front bumper hitting flesh and bone. My right foot slammed the brake pedal. The car stopped just short of an airborne boy, maybe 12 or 13, levitating a few inches above the pavement as his unzipped nylon school bag launched itself from his shoulder and spewed notebooks, pencils and personal effects all over the street.

The kid lay sprawled in a heap on the pavement. A car door slammed somewhere off to my left, and his mother was kneeling beside him, crooning and fussing, her face a mask of incredulous fury completely at odds with her tender ministrations. And then sirens came speeding toward us up the avenue.

As the mother stood behind the ambulance watching them shove the gurney inside, I finally got up the nerve to approach her. She was talking in Spanish with a man who had come over from the auto body shop across from the school. "*Lo siento, señora,*" I said.

"*Lo siento mucho.* I'm very sorry." She wouldn't even look at me. The man from the body shop wasn't so reticent. "I seen it, man," he snarled. "You seen him and you just keep going." And I thought, yes, that's exactly what it must have looked like.

"I just didn't see him," I admitted, which was true. The officer didn't ask me anything about that, or even issue me a ticket. He simply said the kid shouldn't have jaywalked in front of my car, which was also true.

The next few weeks, I spent a lot of time in my apartment, only leaving home for errands I could accomplish on foot. I tried taking the car out one more time to the neighborhood laundromat. But even that short trip unnerved me. So, finally facing facts, I put the car up for sale and surrendered my driver's license for a California ID card.

No one ever contacted me about the accident. I felt justified in assuming—thankfully—that the boy wasn't hurt too badly. But still, every time I think about it, my hands remember the weird, rubber shock of the impact through the steering wheel, and I see the whole thing all over again. I especially remember the look on the mother's face. Some things, some of us learn only the hard way.

Lo siento, señora. Lo siento mucho.[78]

You may be fortunate enough to avoid a tragedy such as this. However, if there is even a chance that such a thing could happen because you are overconfident in your capabilities, then you need to take a step back. Even with perfect sight and quick reactions, people have accidents. There is no good reason to take a chance on hurting yourself or someone else when there are available options.

BiOptic driving

About half of the fifty states allow restricted driving by visually impaired people using a device called a BiOptic telescope.[79] This small telescope is mounted directly on one or both lenses of the driver's prescribed spectacles. It is usually set above and to the side of the axis of vision, but may be affixed elsewhere, depending upon the driver's requirements.

A BiOptic telescope is for periodic use when close-up spotting is necessary, such as reading a street sign. It is not intended for continuous viewing, and it takes practice to use efficiently. More information about BiOptic driving may be obtained from the BiOptic Driving Network at www.biopticdriving.org or by calling (413) 638-6941.

What is the law?

If you have trouble deciding for yourself about driving, the law may help you make up your mind. Your doctor should be aware of the regulations in your state and may even notify the Department of Motor Vehicles (DMV) about your condition.

The vision criteria for approving a driver's license vary slightly from state to state. Here are typical requirements:

Minimum uncorrected visual acuity of 20/40 for unrestricted license and minimum of 20/50 for a restricted license.

Persons with binocular vision and visual acuity of 20/60 restricted to daytime driving only. Doctor's report required.

Monocular persons need 20/40 in the fellow eye.

Visual acuity of 20/70 in the better eye if worse eye
is 20/200 or better. Acuity of 20/40 if worse eye is
worse than 20/200.

Field of vision must be 140 degrees for a person with
vision in both eyes and 105 degrees for a person with
vision in only one eye.

These criteria were gathered from several states to
serve as an example of the most common requirements.
To learn the regulations for your state, contact your
local DMV.

Some experts feel that more areas of testing should
enter into the licensure decision. These tests might include identification of central scotomas, detection of
eye movement disorders, and contrast sensitivity. All of
these vision factors enter into a person's ability to drive
safely. They should, according to some, be considered
along with acuity, visual field, **depth perception,** and
color perception. The bottom line is:

> Driving is a privilege, not a right. A wise person
> knows when it is time to make the road a little safer
> by staying out from behind the wheel.

Alternatives to driving

The Americans with Disabilities Act (ADA) of 1990,
Title II, requires that acceptable alternative transportation be available in every area of the country for people
who are disabled due to visual impairment. According to
several state surveys, acceptable accommodations for
the visually impaired should include:

Accessible, identifiable, and safe waiting areas
Verbal identification of stops and destinations
Tickets and schedules in Braille
Door-to-door service (not just curb-to-curb)
Employees trained in needs of the visually impaired
Assistance in boarding and unboarding
Availability (bus runs at least every 30 minutes)
Adequate number of vehicles
Adequate number and design of routes
Adequate and convenient hours of operation
Service during evenings and weekends
Availability of intercity routes (from town to town)
Fares and fees in line with local economy
Allowance for short stops of less than an hour
Reliable, on-time service

MD Support maintains a searchable national database for locating such transportation services and the accommodations they provide. More than fifteen hundred alternative transportation services have been identified so far in the United States. Such services include the following types:

Local transit bus system (travels throughout your local area)
Commuter bus system (travels between your area and a nearby city or town)
Light rail, rapid rail, or subway system
Commuter train service
Commuter vanpool service
Carpool matching service
Taxi service
Paratransit system (which operates alongside a public

transportation system to provide special amenities. These services may also be provided by private companies or nonprofit organizations.)
Local organization with volunteer drivers
Over-the-road bus (like Greyhound)
Intercity train service (like Amtrak)
Ferry or water taxi
Service providers (Medicaid/Medicare, supported employment rides)

Another source for contact information is "Supplemental Transportation Programs for Seniors," which may be found on the Internet at www.seniordrivers.org.

Most alternative transportation services are located in or near large cities. This means that if you live in a small town or isolated rural area, you may have trouble finding such amenities. That is when you may have to depend upon friends and family members. Here is what AMD community member Charlie Zell had to say about that:

> When you could drive, you may have called upon the three A's of successful alternative transportation for help. Today when you need help finding a ride, you should remember the three A's: Attitude, Attitude, and Attitude. If you do not have a good attitude, you may have difficulties in getting a ride.
>
> Nobody enjoys being around an old grump. Sure we all have our problems, but do not burden your driver with them. We also need to remember that, just because we have a vision handicap, nobody owes us

any special favors. Here are some specific suggestions for developing your own transportation system:

Be friendly and courteous. Always thank your driver for the ride.

Get to know your neighbors. The more you know and the better you know them, the better chance you may have of finding a ride. Learn their habits and routines, and coordinate your activities with theirs.

Plan ahead and be organized. Nobody should be considered as being at your call or beckoning at a moment's notice.

Reward your driver's thoughtfulness by offering to pay for a tank of gas, buying lunch, giving appropriate gifts or cards to remember birthdays, holidays, and special events.

Spread the business around. Do not call on a person too frequently. It is also a good idea to have an ace up your sleeve. That is a person you rarely call upon but who may be able to help when you are in dire need.

Avoid criticizing the person's driving or the particular route they choose to take. If you don't like it, keep quiet, find somebody else, or stay home.

Don't forget: Attitude, Attitude, Attitude.[80]

It isn't easy to give up driving and depend upon others for help, but remember: part of your TASK force is "Adaptability." It *can* be done, so if it *should* be done, make it your responsibility before someone else has to make the decision for you. You will be admired and respected for your wisdom in doing so.

IN A SENTENCE:

> *Driving a vehicle is a convenience—maybe even a necessity—but it isn't worth a life. You can develop your own transportation system with some thoughtful organization, planning, and social interaction.*

MONTH 5

Protect Yourself

FOCAL POINTS:

- *Learn your rights under the law.*
- *Beware of solicitations for donations from companies with which you are unfamiliar.*

AT THIS time, you may feel vulnerable. The fact is that you *are* more vulnerable than usual. Both your emotional and your physical health can be weakened by the trauma of vision loss. Unfortunately, this can cause you to make decisions and judgments that you would not normally make. Month 5 will empower you with the information you may need to keep you out of potentially awkward or hazardous situations.

Your legal rights under the Americans with Disabilities Act (ADA)

The Americans with Disabilities Act (ADA) is a federal law enacted by Congress in 1990. It protects all disabled persons against discrimination by public and private employers, programs, services, facilities, and transportation.

The ADA defines disability as "a physical or mental impairment that substantially limits one or more of the major life activities of such individual."[81] If you are losing sight, and you still need to remain in the work force, you should realize that you have the right to reasonable accommodations in order for you to function efficiently and effectively on the job. You can expect your employer, for example, to provide adequate lighting in your work area. And if you use a computer, magnification software and a text reader program are not unreasonable expectations. If you work for a company that has fifteen or more employees, or if you work for the state or local government, your rights are protected by law under the Americans with Disabilities Act.

Basically, the ADA states that if you are qualified to perform essential job functions except for limitations caused by your vision, the employer must consider whether you could perform those functions with reasonable accommodation. "Reasonable accommodation" might mean altering your work environment, modifying equipment, or even reassigning you to another position for which you are qualified.

For more information about your rights under the Americans with Disabilities Act, contact the Equal

Employment Opportunity Commission. The information they provide is available in standard and large print, on audiocassette, in Braille, and on computer disk. Their contact information is:

> U.S. Equal Employment Opportunity
>   Commission
> 1801 L Street, NW
> Washington, DC 20507
> Telephone: (202) 663-4900
> Web site: www.eeoc.gov

How to avoid charity rip-offs

You have been recently diagnosed. The sense of urgency you feel can make you particularly vulnerable in your earnest desire to fight back with everything at your disposal, including your pocketbook. It is, therefore, important that you let your natural street smarts remain in control.

Wherever you find people who are affected by incurable diseases, you will find others trying to relieve them of their money. Often hiding under the guise of nonprofit charitable organizations and carefully following all of the requirements imposed by law, they present a façade of benevolence, warning of impending danger, and then beg "as much as you can afford" and "without delay" to help them eliminate it. Whether or not the danger is real is beside the issue. They only need to make enough people believe it.

Using scare tactics, their appeal is usually loaded with frightening rhetoric such as, "You may become a victim of this life-threatening disease," or "Macular degeneration

will stalk you and shatter your life!" This is often followed by such comforting assurances as "Act now, and
your donation can stop this crippling enemy." Not only
does language such as this often walk a thin line of truth,
but it is also designed to inflame the emotions of the
solicitors' target audiences, the majority of whom are
either candidates for or are already affected by the disease.

These tactics are unconscionable, and they are so successful that huge amounts of money are being pock-
eted. One organization that uses this approach, for
example, reports annual revenues in the millions, but
contributes only about 15 percent to program activities.
The acceptable standard is at least 65 percent.[82]

Certainly there are worthy causes that deserve public
support, but how does one determine which organizations are aboveboard and which are simply wolves in
sheep's clothing? The following information may help to
answer that question. What should you do if you receive a solicitation letter or phone call from an unfamiliar charity? A solicitation should be ignored if . . .

It causes you to feel pressured into sending money
immediately.
It causes you to feel afraid or unusually uncomfortable
in any way.
It makes promises that seem far-fetched.
It promotes the sender's organization as the only hope.
It is sprinkled with patronizing remarks.
It requests personal financial information.
It announces that you have won a prize, that you have
been specially selected, or that you need to honor a
donation pledge that you don't remember making.

Phone calls are harder to ignore than letters, because gracious people find it difficult to hang up. The easiest way to end such conversations is to say, "I'm sorry, but I do not make financial commitments by phone. Please mail the information to me, and I will be happy to look it over." A legitimate organization will do so, and you have bought yourself some time to think more about it at your leisure—something an unethical solicitor will not want you to do.

If you feel that you are in doubt about a particular organization, contact the Better Business Bureau Wise Giving Alliance, which can tell you whether or not a charity meets certain standards. Here is how to get in touch:

BBB Wise Giving Alliance
4200 Wilson Blvd., Suite 800
Arlington, VA 22203
Telephone: (703) 276-0100
Web site: www.give.org

Knowledge is a powerful weapon, and it can be our lack of it that will allow people to take advantage. The more people there are who have the right information, the less harm unethical solicitors can do, and the more money there will be for truly deserving charities.

IN A SENTENCE:

Low vision will not turn you into a victim if you know the facts and where to get help.

Straight Talk about Cope-ability

FOCAL POINTS:

▶ *How strong is your cope-ability?*
▶ *Your strength comes from within.*

COPE-ABILITY is something everyone needs at some time or another in the course of life, particularly when experiencing loss of eyesight. It is something deep inside that waits until it is needed. When summoned, it rises to the surface, ready to offer comfort in the knowledge that everything will be all right. But what is it? Is it part of the original human hardware, or does it need to be built? If it needs to be built, then what materials are required?

Some people seem to be born with cope-ability. Compare different babies. Some of them just deal with the stresses of life as a newborn. No one shows them how, they just do it. Most babies, however, melt down several times a day for no discernible reason. They are fragile, insecure little eggs, and their emotional insides are easily scrambled. Some emotionally labile people survive through adulthood by depending upon family and friends for support. That may be good in the short term, but most people manage eventually to slap together their own specially designed cope-abilities using materials gathered from living the greater part of a life. And usually, those who have it the toughest survive the best. Take those people at your fortieth class reunion, for example. Ted, the asthmatic boy who had to stay in at recess, is now a respected college professor. Wilma, who worked every day after school to help support her family, now owns a thriving company. Did they make lemonade out of lemons? More likely, they sold the lemons and drank water instead. They "made do."

"Making do" means facing a situation and using the materials at hand to make the best of it, simply because there is no other sensible option. You are losing your central vision. You can do nothing about it at this time except to maintain your physical and psychological health until the problem can be fixed. It's time to make do with the materials at hand: low vision devices, technology, support opportunities, and adaptive solutions. These materials are plentiful and available, but it is up to you to gather them. That's where your cope-ability comes in. So how "cope-able" are you?

Your cope-ability score

Below is a list of thirty character strengths that have proved to be helpful to those who are walking the AMD road. Find your cope-ability score by checking those characteristics that apply most of the time to you.

Your cope-ability strengths

[ ] You deal with problems one at a time, rather than letting them pile up.

[ ] You compose lists of positives and negatives when a tough decision has to be made.

[ ] You identify escape routes in case plans go awry.

[ ] You practice techniques such as counting to ten or controlled breathing during times of stress.

[ ] You let go of thoughts that really don't matter.

[ ] You use yesterday's lessons to plan for tomorrow.

[ ] You enjoy the present, because you realize that it is *always* the present.

[ ] You expect the best, but prepare for the worst.

[ ] You give yourself the gift of time.

[ ] You never say what you think until you've thought.

[ ] You don't sweat the small stuff, but you work hard on the big stuff.

[ ] You maintain a bit of knowledgeable cynicism.

[ ] You believe that miracles can happen.

[ ] You let your enthusiasm show.

[ ] You look for hope in everything.

[ ] You love and laugh a lot.

[ ] You make no excuses.

[ ] You lay no blame.

[ ] You accept responsibility for your own actions.

[ ] You look for possibilities inside yourself.

[ ] You are your own best friend, cheerleader, and entertainment director.

[ ] You get plenty of rejuvenating sleep.

[ ] You eat and drink well.

[ ] You exercise.

[ ] You reward yourself for little successes.

[ ] You forgive yourself for little failures.

[ ] If you feel as though your glass is half empty, you get a smaller glass.

[ ] You think of strangers as your friends.

[ ] You embrace change while respecting tradition.

[ ] You laugh and cry enthusiastically, because you know how healthy that can be.

Total checked: ___/30

Scoring:

30/30 You should think about starting a talk show. The world needs to learn from you.

22–29 You will be successful at this low vision thing. Congratulations!

15–21 You will do fine if you can raise your score as soon as possible. Make that your most immediate goal.

8–14 You have some work to do. Start with the easiest to change, then build on those successes.

0–7 You are as delicate as an eggshell. Hopefully, this book will give you the strength you need to cope with the challenges of AMD. If you cannot get your score up to at least 20, please consider talking to someone who can help you sort out your thoughts and the direction you want to take.

A Message from the AMD Community

Dear Friends,

I recognize that I still view visual impairment as a weakness. I wonder why, as I have learned that most people with visual impairment are stronger than those who have never faced adversity.

We meet so many people on MDList who have found ways to overcome so many challenges. Why then do we, who are new to vision difficulties, see ourselves as less than we were, prior to the eye condition? I will spend some time today contemplating on this matter.

We do, however, have choices. We can choose to let this condition get us down and feel like victims, or we can choose to feel empowered and get on with providing the best quality of life possible for ourselves.

I go to the gym for strength training. I am frustrated, because I have a problem setting the equipment and can't read the computer screens on some of the machines. I don't discuss this with my trainer. I just wait for him to set everything.

He was telling me he has a client who has been blind since childhood. If you could see this building, you would be impressed that she even finds her way into the bowels of the university. She not only finds her way, she sets her own machines and no longer needs assistance to find her way around the busy room full of various moving equipment.

The trainer was only making conversation with me, but I felt like a whiner.

On Friday, I will set my own weights.

Sharon N.

Helpful ideas for coping with low vision

Regardless of your score, there are things you can do every day to make your life easier. These ideas were contributed by people who have AMD, so you can trust the ideas to be practical and worthwhile. Like the earlier list of tips for adapting your home, these suggestions will help improve your quality of life. This list focuses on ways that you can cope with low vision on a personal level.

IN THE KITCHEN:

Record recipes on a tape recorder. When you are cooking or using the recipe, you can use the pause button between tasks.

Shop online or have groceries delivered.

Cook prepared foods or frozen vegetables when in a hurry. (Keep in mind, of course, the high sodium and fat content of many prepared foods. High fat content is bad for the circulation of the blood in the retina. High sodium intakes can also be hazardous to your overall health.)

Ask the butcher to quarter the chicken or cube the beef for you.

Don't hesitate to touch or knead food with your hands, as long as they are clean.

To pour a liquid, use your finger to align the edges of the containers. Raise the edge of the pouring container slightly over the edge of the receiving container. Listen for the sound as the container fills, feel the weight, estimate the time. Alternatively, purchase a liquid level indicator that beeps when the container is nearing full.

For easy cleanup and neatness, use a cookie tray to prepare food on. Grate or chop directly into a bowl.

Use bowls with nonslip bases or place a nonslip mat on the countertop.

Consider purchasing a Stir Chef automatic pot stirrer and a pan holder.

Use the end of a utensil to locate meat in the pan before flipping.

Purchase a tactile or talking timer.

To get organized:

Buy different colored bins and boxes to organize receipts, office supplies, personal papers, computer stuff, etc.

When withdrawing cash from the bank, take white envelopes with the dollar amounts clearly marked.

Put receipts in little baggies to ensure that they don't get lost in your purse or pocket.

Organizing with bags:

Organizing with cloth bags diminishes the frustration of looking for items, as well as helping you avoid being late because you just can't find something. Look for plain dollar-store bags in a variety of colors. They even have a change purse attached. These are also relatively simple to make if you know someone who can sew. Velcro closures are handy. Here are some good uses for bags:

- A bag for your lamp, an extension cord, large playing cards, tissue, money, and other necessities for going to bridge games.
- A bag for your exercise class needs: member card, exercise instructions, lock and shoes.
- A Grandpa or Grandma bag with a toy, a book, etc., for going to quiet places with grandchildren.
- A bag with tools for meetings. This includes extra dollars for just in case. It also includes extra house keys.
- A bag with everything you need if you are going to be sitting and waiting somewhere: handwork, a portable tape or CD player, earphones, a book and lighted magnifier, etc.

For the ladies: makeup and grooming

Makeup: Subtle is best with all makeup, but using it gives you a lift. The bonus is that, with practice, you are able to apply makeup anywhere at any time and get it right. Once you learn how to apply makeup with limited vision, you'll learn that no mirror is really required. The tricky part is not so much in applying it, but whether it is applied evenly and balanced. This can be more accurately done by using your finger in place of a brush for blush and eye shadow. (One woman with AMD has suggested using liquid coloring on your upper eyelid, because you can feel it going on.) And as for eyeliner, just forget it.

After using toner and moisturizer, hang on to the pad you used for the toner. Apply powder eye shadow with your finger and, after using the mascara, take the moistened pad and carefully wipe around your eyes just to remove any signs of powder or slight touches of mascara. This will give you a great feeling of confidence that nothing is smudged!

As you practice, try to have someone there who will give you continuous feedback. If no one is around, use a magnifying mirror and a strong light to check for yourself. After a while, you will get the feel for it, but it never hurts to have an honest friend check you out once in a while.

Hair: Call your hairdresser ahead of time, and schedule an appointment for when she won't be too busy. Let her know that you would like a style that is easy to manage. A good cut and a few hair care hints work wonders.

Feet and hands: Don't turn up your nose at a pedicure and/or a manicure. You need these to ensure good health. Don't hesitate to ask for a manicure for a birthday or holiday gift.

Clothes: No one wants to leave the house wearing dirty garments, and you might tend to spill more food than you would think. Have a trusted individual help you keep a close watch: someone who will be truthful when pointing out unsightly stains or spills. If you can't always have someone to help, then follow this simple rule: if in doubt, throw it in the laundry.

Shoes: People with low vision tend to trip and bang their toes, so tips of shoes will deteriorate faster. A loose sole could cause you a nasty fall. Feel the toe for separation from the sole. Slippery leather soles are an added hazard, so buy rubber soles. Tie your shoes together in pairs when storing them, and keep them in their original boxes for easier identification.

IN THE BATHROOM:

Put your hair dryer, curling iron, brush, and other related supplies in a one-handled basket that fits under the sink.

In a washable open container place a clean face cloth, toothbrush, etc. Clean and/or replace the contents on a regular basis.

A night-light is imperative. Sudden full lighting in the night can be painful and may temporarily blind you.

Use plastic pill dispensers that are clearly and securely labeled. It is so easy to take the wrong medicine. It is a good idea to have your pharmacist mark the lids of your medications clearly and in large print before you pay for them. The pharmacist will also remove the safety cap for you if you have no small children in the house. It's easy to do: Just pry out the inner cap and discard it. The remaining cap becomes the lid. With some bottles, you can simply flip the cap over for the easy-to-open version.

WHEN TRAVELING:

Let your carrier, whether it be airline, train, or bus, know you have low vision.

Pack items in see through bags. I use the bags off linens. Zip-lock bags are also great. Use tissue paper as well. Stockings/socks in one bag, underwear in another, ties in one, and jewelry in another. Layer matched outfits with tissue between. I found that wrapping outfits in tissue the way they do in department stores reduces wrinkles.

Take a placemat, bright green or white, and lay out your morning needs on it. This also works at home. At night, put your watch, etc., on a placemat so they are easily found.

Put travel documents in a folder and then in a bag.

Never bring more than you can carry.

Money is a nuisance, so use a credit or debit card if possible. This avoids having to make the exchange and or change.

If you are traveling alone, count the doors from the elevator to the room. Have a porter take the time to show you the elevator buttons and note them verbally, out loud.

Carry a flashlight or a lighted magnifier for reading restaurant menus.

If the restaurant is too dark to see what is on your plate, order finger food, such as a sandwich, chicken, or ribs.

If eating in restaurants is too much of a challenge, room service can be a great option.

Always have a meeting point in case you get separated from your companion. This is also good for a shopping date. Have your companion wear a color you can see.

Tag your bag with a bright ribbon or strap that you can see.

Keep your valuables hidden in a secret pocket on your person, not in your purse. This is especially important if you can be identified by strangers as visually impaired, such as by using a white cane.

Leave a copy of all your documents (including bank cards) with a family member in case you lose yours.

Travelers checks are handy and safe, but signing them is a challenge. Get a heavy piece of paper, Mylar, or cardboard ahead of time, and make a template by cutting it to the size of the check. Then cut out the five individual blocks where you need to write, specifically: the date, the name of the recipient, the dollar amount, the spelled-out amount, and your signature. Keep the template in your checkbook, and mistakes will become a thing of the past.

OTHER SUGGESTIONS

How do you tell the front of a garment from the back? With pajamas, for example, it isn't always easy to tell. If there are hanger loops, tie a knot in the left or front loop. Sew a spare button in the left front hem. Even a French knot works fine. Being consistent is the key.

For safety when out walking, wear brightly colored outer garments, such as a lightweight white windbreaker in warmer weather and a red jacket when it snows.

Keep different denominations of folding money in separate compartments of your billfold. Another good idea: fold each denomination differently or bend down a different corner to mark $1, $5, $10, and $20 bills.

Hang a sign in your kitchen warning anyone who moves something to replace it to its original location. Knowing the location of your stuff is critical to both your safety and your sanity.

Have all of your door locks fixed so that you need only one key to get in and out. Give a spare key to a family member and another to a trusted neighbor.

Have motion-detector lights installed at entrances, both inside and out.

Call your phone company about free directory assistance and operator-assisted dialing. Your doctor should be able to help you with the approval and application process.

Get rid of scatter rugs and loose carpets. If you have a favorite rug with a design you just love, consider hanging it on the wall. It will last much longer there, and you can see it better!

Detours

Isn't it amazing? You set out in life with an empty bag and a vision of a straight, smoothly paved road, along which you plan to travel unhindered into your future. But sometimes barriers block your way. You then have a choice to either give up the journey or shoulder your bag and take the detours.

That's the amazing part: there will always be detours, which may take you in some very interesting directions. And every time you return to the main road from one of those adventures, your bag will be a little heavier with the stuff you have picked up: souvenirs, hitchhikers, treasures, even some trash. It's all in there, and good or bad, it is a unique collection.

You may be hesitant right now, but, hopefully, your fear of the unknown will not stop you from taking the detours, because that's where you will find the brave people. And when you finally reach the end of your journey, you will be able to hand your bag to the person walking behind you and say, "I wouldn't have missed that for all the green tea in China!"

Every experience starts out as an unknown. It's part of the human spirit to explore it, learn about it, and adapt to it, and that's how progress is made. Learning to cope with a detour like low vision, as frightening as it may seem at first, can be a growing experience that surpasses anything you have ever accomplished. Millions have already walked the road, and millions more are walking it now with you. It is undoubtedly not the direction you intended to go, but now it's there in front of you. You may as well embrace the challenge and see what adventures lie ahead.

And as you move forward, remember that visual impairment does not define you. You are still the person who started out on this journey a few decades ago. This is simply another collection of interesting stuff for your bag.

A Message from the AMD Community: Laughter Is Good Medicine

Lord Byron wrote, "Always laugh when you can. It is cheap medicine." After paying the deductible on your eye care insurance and wading through some of the heavy stuff in this book, a cheap laugh would probably hit the spot right about now.

I feel my life is all a blur:
I cannot tell a him from her.
I once approached a garbage pail,
And thought it an attractive male.

And since I am a friendly soul,
I wave and smile at every pole.
And this is just the normal state
Of a macular degenerate.

Marion G.

IN A SENTENCE:

> *How well you travel this road depends upon how well you cope with its hills, valleys, twists, and turns. Following in the footsteps of those who have gone before will help to make your journey easier.*

HALF-YEAR **MILESTONE**

You are halfway to a good understanding of a disease that affects more than 8.5 million people in the United States alone. Hopefully, you are feeling the confidence that comes with knowledge and support. Here is what you have learned these past few months:

○ WHAT TO ASK (AND NOT ASK) YOUR DOCTOR.

○ WAYS TO HELP YOU NAVIGATE YOUR EVERYDAY LIFE.

○ THE IMPORTANT ISSUES INVOLVED IN DRIVING WITH VISUAL IMPAIRMENT.

○ HOW TO AVOID BEING TAKEN AD-VANTAGE OF BECAUSE OF YOUR CONDITION.

The Art and Practice of Eccentric Viewing

FOCAL POINT:

▸ *You can learn to read and see better with your peripheral vision.*

ECCENTRIC VIEWING is a technique used by people with central vision loss. It is a method by which the person looks slightly away from the subject in order to view it peripherally with another area of the visual field. This is similar to looking slightly away from an object at night in order to see it better. By doing so, the viewer is allowing the rod cells in the peripheral field to take over for the cone cells in the central field. Rod cells are better than cone cells for viewing in dim light.

In normal light, images are focused directly onto the macula, or the very center of the retina, where the cone cells are most dense. The cone cells are responsible for both color and fine-detail vision. When they lose that ability, the rod cells can be taught to take over to some extent. With proper training, concentrated practice, and proper adaptations, these less acute areas can act as a reasonable substitute.[83]

The biological task of eccentric viewing is complex. It requires your eyes and brain to learn a new method of seeing, which means developing new habits and skills. This can usually be accomplished over a period of about six visits with a trained low vision therapist. In addition, home practice is important for supplementing the training and speeding the progress. It is difficult to self-teach eccentric viewing, because it can be frustrating. An experienced, observant professional can help alleviate frustration by offering you new approaches when others may not be working.

Remember that training in eccentric viewing will not improve the condition of the retina. You may feel that your vision has improved as a result, but that is simply because you have maximized your existing vision.

Your first step in the training is identifying the blind areas (scotomas). After that, techniques are introduced that help you learn to work around those areas. These techniques include tracing, identifying cards, and other methods used to improve reading and writing skills. Your detail vision will not be fully regained by eccentric viewing training, but it can be greatly improved when coupled with appropriate magnification devices, good lighting, and enhanced contrast (the "Three Bs" introduced in

Day 5: Bigger, Brighter, and Bolder). The level of reading ability that you can attain is determined in large part by your visual condition and determination.

For training in eccentric viewing, contact a low vision rehabilitation center. These can be located in the phone book under "Rehabilitation Services," by asking a low vision specialist, or by contacting the appropriate state agency listed in Appendix A.

Perhaps you would like to take on the challenge of developing eccentric viewing skills on your own. Here is a self-training program developed by Jennifer Galbraith, OD, MS, and used successfully in her practice at Rebman Eye Care in Elizabethtown, Pennsylvania.

Self-training exercises

Following are four sets of three images for the purpose of practicing eccentric vision. The sizes of the images grow progressively smaller with each set.

The assumption is that you have a central scotoma (blind spot) in either or both eyes. Begin by propping this book up in good lighting and moving five to ten feet away. Look directly at the letter A in Exercise 1, making it disappear or become very blurred. Then look slightly to the side, above, or below the letter, making it reappear. Be sure to keep your head still.

Once you can read the letter, hold your eye in that position, called your **preferred retinal locus (PRL)**, as long as possible. When you feel that you can comfortably see the letter eccentrically, then move on to Exercise 2, and repeat the process. Take your time. If you have difficulty seeing the letter after five or ten minutes, bookmark the page and return to it later. Your brain needs time to adjust to this new way of looking at things. Eccentric viewing is not an easy skill to develop, but don't give up. With patience and daily practice, it will eventually become second nature.

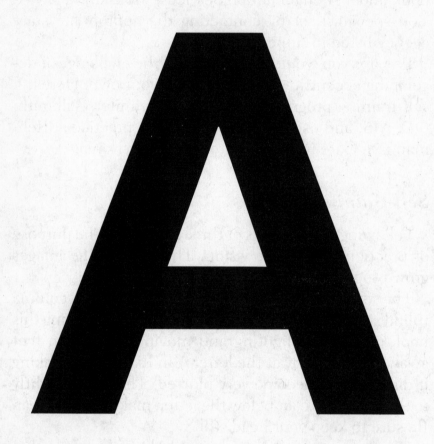

Exercise 1

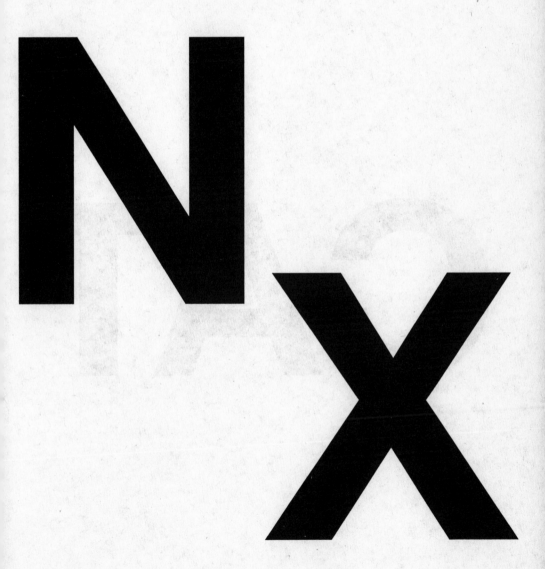

Exercise 2

CAT

Exercise 3

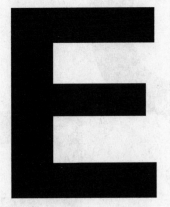

Exercise 4

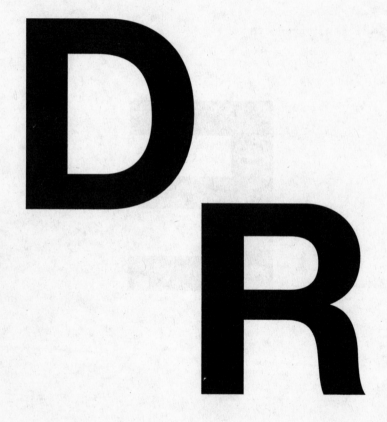

Exercise 5

PIG

Exercise 6

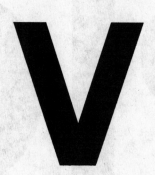

Exercise 7

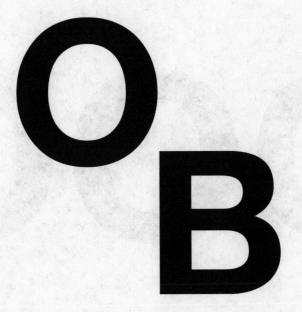

Exercise 8

DOG

Exercise 9

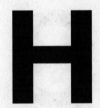

Exercise 10

S

Exercise 11

HAD

Exercise 12

Learning to use your peripheral vision will help you in many ways other than reading. Eccentric viewing is an important skill that can help maximize your vision and make every facet of daily living easier. These exercises are a very basic introduction to the skill and practice of eccentric viewing. For further instruction, an excellent reading workshop is included in Dr. Lylas Mogk's book *Macular Degeneration: The Complete Guide to Saving and Maximizing Your Sight* (see Month 12: "Further Reading"). You will also find that working with someone else will make the task easier. You may want to contact your local low vision rehabilitation center to acquire the guidance of a personal low vision therapist. (See Appendix A, or ask your doctor for contact information.)

IN A SENTENCE:

You can improve your reading ability using the "Three Bs" (Bigger, Brighter, Bolder) in combination with training and practice in eccentric viewing, either on your own or with professional guidance.

Your Success Is Mostly Up to You

PLEASE TAKE a few minutes to reflect on three important questions: Are you going to allow AMD to put the brakes on your life? Are you willing to look for workable alternatives to good eyesight? Will you let AMD have a negative affect on who you are?

The two basic types of visually impaired people are those who are successful and those who are not. Some people (maybe you) even seem to *thrive* as a result of their impairment. Adversity seems to bring out the best in some people, but why not everybody? Why does one person move on while another gives up? Is it possible to change?

To begin exploring possible answers to those questions, here are transcripts of real conversations with two people with AMD.

A conversation with Millie

MILLIE: I hate trying to read menus in dark restaurants. Why can't they turn on the lights?

DAN: Do you have a lighted magnifier?

MILLIE: Yes, but I can't use it.

DAN: Wrong magnification?

MILLIE: Dead batteries.

DAN: Why don't you replace them?

MILLIE: I can't get to the store.

DAN: But you get to the restaurant.

MILLIE: My daughter takes me.

DAN: Could your daughter pick up some batteries for you?

MILLIE: I suppose so.

DAN: Then you could read the menu?

MILLIE: Yes.

DAN: And the restaurant could continue to use nice soft lighting.

MILLIE: I suppose so.

A conversation with Phil

PHIL: I can't see the television anymore.

DAN: How large is the screen?

PHIL: I can't afford one of those big ones.

DAN: Okay. Where do you sit to watch it?

PHIL: In my recliner across the room.

DAN: Have you tried binocular glasses?

PHIL: Can't afford them.

DAN: If I get you some, would you wear them?

PHIL: They hurt my nose.

DAN: Okay. Have you tried sitting closer?

PHIL: Can't move the chair. Bad back.

DAN: If I come over and move it, do you think that would solve your problem?

PHIL: Might work. What would that cost me?

DAN: A cup of hot tea.

PHIL: Don't have any tea.

DAN: Do you have a cup?

PHIL: Yep.

DAN: I'll bring the tea. How about tonight?

PHIL: Wanta stay and watch the game?

DAN: Sure.

PHIL: See you at six.

Acceptance of personal responsibility is difficult enough. Then, when disability enters the equation, the willingness to transfer responsibility to others is often magnified. This was the position in which Millie and Phil found themselves in. The burden of low vision made the world a more difficult place, and they didn't recognize the power they had to make it better. That was a new way of thinking that hadn't occurred to them. While loss of sight can often bring insight, it can also skew a person's perspective if they are looking for answers in the wrong places.

It is hard to accept that no one is to blame for your diminished vision. Not only is there nowhere to lay the blame, but the highly visual world you live in cannot, in all fairness, be expected to meet you more than halfway. The restaurant provides enough light for Millie to reach her table and for most people to read by. Millie must then accept the responsibility for taking care of her personal needs beyond that.

Phil owns a chair and a television. Companies offer low

vision devices to help him span the distance between the two. If, however, current technology cannot help, then Phil's challenge is to experiment with ways to solve the problem. He might enjoy listening to the game on a radio, for example, or he could simply move closer to the television. Why didn't he think of that himself? Because as a new VIP, he was unaccustomed to thinking outside of the box and seeing the obvious. Here is Edna's story, which shows what can be accomplished when one simply steps back and lets common sense prevail.

Edna's story

All I wanted to do was iron my blouse for church. So I found the ironing board and my old steam iron with no difficulty (because I have learned to be very organized) and set them up in the kitchen. After plugging in the iron by feeling for the socket and somehow not electrocuting myself, I discovered that the reservoir was empty. As the iron heated up, I filled a measuring cup at the sink and returned to perform what used to be a simple procedure.

I never thought pouring water could be such a challenge. That was a tiny little hole, and I had to hit it directly with no central vision. It would have been easy if I had a funnel, but who owns a funnel anymore? I guess I could have made one out of paper, but that would have meant finding paper, scissors, and tape. This shouldn't be so difficult, and I don't have the time!

I tried making a funnel out of my fingers and only made a mess. That's when I decided to just wear the blouse wrinkled. Who would care, anyway? "I'm an old blind lady, for Pete's sake," I said aloud. "What do they expect?"

I started to cry. And that made me mad. And the madder I got, the harder I cried. Then a big tear dropped onto the blouse, and I flashed back to my mother sprinkling water on my pinafore with her fingers.

"How stupid of me!" I thought, and within an hour, I was at church with a freshly ironed blouse done the old-fashioned way.

Edna has probably always been a positive person. That outlook is now what carries her through the daily challenges of vision loss. Millie and Phil may not be in the habit of thinking this way, but maybe it's not too late to change. Low vision does not identify you. If your glass has always been half full, then AMD will probably not change that. If, on the other hand, your glass has always been half *empty,* maybe it's time to get a smaller glass.

Bill used to sit in his backyard and watch the sun set over the mountains. However, AMD took the mountains away. Instead of grieving over that, he and his wife now take more frequent trips to the mountains, giving them more time together and giving him something to look forward to at least once a month. The rest of the month, Bill enjoys watching the sun set over his vegetable garden, which, he says, "is a heck of a lot easier to see."

So Bill got himself a smaller glass. His expectations of himself, therefore, are no higher than his abilities, and he is a happy man. When people think about Bill (and they often do), they don't think of him as "Bill, the guy with low vision," they think of him as "Bill, the guy who makes us smile."

You've probably seen those optical illusions that require you to view them in a different way in order for you to see the obvious. You know, those pictures that make you exclaim, "Oh, *now* I see it!" Well, problems caused by visual impairment can be just as mystifying or clearly solvable, depending upon how you perceive them.

Four common challenges are listed below. Assuming that no one is around to help, which of the two possible responses do you think would be most appropriate?

CHALLENGE: You are waiting to cross a busy street, and you can't see the "walk" signal.

Choice #1: Turn around, go home, and write a letter to city hall requesting that they install audio signals.

Choice #2: Watch and listen to the traffic. When it starts to move on the street parallel to you, it's time to cross. When you get back home, write that letter.

CHALLENGE: The bus driver isn't announcing the stops, so you don't know when to get off.

Choice #1: If you ever get home, write to the bus company requesting that their drivers announce all stops.

Choice #2: Ask the driver to notify you when your stop comes. Sit near him, and if necessary, ask at each stop. When you get home, write your letter.

CHALLENGE: When the store clerk gives you your change, you suspect that she is trying to cheat you again by returning a five-dollar bill instead of a ten.

Choice #1: Not wanting to be confrontational, leave quietly, go home, and write a letter to the store manager about the incident.

Choice #2: Ask the clerk to break the bill into ten ones. Smirking rightfully, take your ten dollar bills home and write the letter.

CHALLENGE: The elevator door opens, it's empty, and you can't see whether it's going to go up or down.

Choice #1: Turn around, go home, and write a letter requesting that they install audio elevator systems in their building.

Choice #2: If the elevator is empty, it's probably going your direction (assuming you pressed the correct button). If someone is in it, ask them which way it's going. Then, when you get home . . . well, you know.

This should give you an idea as to how creative thinking can not only be beneficial, it can also make for an interesting day. When you are faced with a challenge, first of all, take in a slow, relaxing breath. There is probably no hurry. Then open your mind to all possibilities, and draw upon the wisdom of your years. You'll probably be pretty impressed with the things you can come up with.

IN A SENTENCE:

> *With a positive attitude and the help of others, you can set the stage for a successful life in spite of low vision.*

Learning from Living: Seeing Well with AMD

FOCAL POINT:

> ▶ *You may be losing some of your sight, but you are not losing your vision.*

Does a visually impaired person have impaired vision?

That sounds like an odd question, but it shines light into the core of an AMD person's self-concept. The answer is found in a close look at the definitions of "visual" and "vision."

The American Heritage Dictionary defines "visual" as something that relates to the sense of sight by means of a visual organ or the visual receptors on the retina.[84] This definition is physiologically based. It leaves no argument that in order to be visual, you must be able to make use of your retina.

The same reference defines "vision" more mystically. "Vision" is more than sight or something that is seen. It is also "intelligent foresight" and "unusual competence in perception." It can even be "a mental image produced by the imagination."[85]

In other words, you need a working retina to be visual, but you could be totally blind and still have vision. That is comforting and absolutely true. It explains why AMD people are called "visually impaired," rather than "vision impaired."

Can you "see" with AMD?

This question is a bit trickier. "Yes," you might answer, "but not well." A little drilling down, however, might provide some interesting insight.

Here are questions based upon the definitions of the words "see" from two different dictionaries.[86] To how many can you respond with a "yes?"Can you . . .

[ ] make sense of things?   [ ] learn?
[ ] assign meanings?   [ ] imagine?
[ ] perceive?   [ ] conceive of ideas?
[ ] become aware?   [ ] live through
[ ] be careful or certain to   experiences?
    do something?   [ ] understand?
[ ] consider?   [ ] observe?
[ ] regard?   [ ] check out?
[ ] deliberate?   [ ] watch?
[ ] decide?   [ ] behold?

[ ] view?   [ ] ascertain?
[ ] discern?   [ ] regard attentively?
[ ] distinguish?   [ ] look after?

If you said "yes" to the majority of them, you obviously
can see in many ways, most of which have nothing to do
with your eyes. And you will be amazed at how much better you can "see" when you allow nonophthalmic viewing to take over.

You have heard of amazing accomplishments by people who are totally blind. Usually, such people are born
blind or become so at a very early age. This causes their
brains to develop alternative neural connections, allowing them to "see" nonvisually. To a sighted person, such
sensory substitutions appear superhuman, but to the
blind person they are nothing more than tools for sur-
vival. These tools can include some (but not necessarily
all) of the following abilities at varying levels of prowess:

musical pitch recognition (from good relative pitch to
    perfect pitch)
memorization (from extraordinary to total recall)
spatial awareness (ability to "hear" or "feel without
    touching" the surrounding space)
highly developed senses of hearing (aural), taste (oral),
    touch (tactile), and smell (olfactory).

Stories are fairly common about blind people who perform amazing feats. Such people play and compose
music, sing arias by memory after a single hearing, and
walk around obstacles that their eyes can't perceive.
Amazing? Why? Because they can't see? Back to that
point in a moment.

Did you know that, by a fully sighted person's standards, your pet pooch is visually impaired? That's right. Fifi (like dogs of every other name) is red/green color-blind, has a central visual acuity somewhere between 20/50 and 20/100, and sees poorly in daylight.[87]

Have you been amazed that Fifi doesn't run into walls? If you haven't been, you probably are now; but you needn't be. She is operating by other senses instead of by sight: not because she is visually impaired, but because she does better this way. If she were to lose her senses of smell and hearing, *then* Fifi would be impaired.

Back to blind people. Ask a congenitally blind child if he is amazing because he can identify where you are standing in the room, and he will probably ask you why you think that's so amazing. He isn't being humble, he really means it. He sees you—just not in the way that you see him. Ask a congenitally blind musician how he can play a piece of music after hearing it only once, and he'll tell you he's reading it—just not like you do. Take the hand of a congenitally blind child when you pass by a stairwell, and she might tell you, "Don't worry. I see it." And she *does* see it—just not like you do.

Actually, what is most amazing about the congenitally blind is that they can live at all in a world designed by ophthalmic people. People who create stairs, sharp corners, stoplights, printed words, color coding, and poles in the middle of nowhere. People who set their clocks by the daylight, judge one another by physical appearance, and communicate through pantomime. People who turn red with embarrassment, blue with the cold, green with envy, and white with fear. People who lower their eyes in shame, stare in defiance, and gaze in awe.

But blind people *do* live in this world, and often

successfully. Thanks to changes in the law, electronic birds chirp when it's safe to cross the street, hills have returned in the form of ramps, bus stops talk, and public signs are in braille. And thanks to the bottomless well of human creativity, the low vision community has descriptive movies, audiobooks, braille, text-to-speech technology, a whole slew of assistive devices, and even personal satellite guidance systems.

So why do some AMD people seem to have such a hard time? Understandably, because they have been "wired" ophthalmically. Pull the plug on a significant part of their vision, and the light goes out on a huge part of their world. If they are then to live successfully as visually impaired people, they first have to admit that they cannot see by conventional means. Then they have to make the effort to rewire themselves, and that may mean seeking professional assistance through low vision rehabilitation.

Most AMD people are senior adults or close to it, and you are probably one of them. The last thing you want to do at this time in your life is start over. Your days of learning are supposed to have been traded by now for days of offering hard-earned wisdom to anyone younger than you whom you can get to sit still and listen.

No wonder AMD is difficult to bear. It wasn't supposed to happen. You don't want to deal with it, and you just want it to go away. Unfortunately, it won't be going away any time soon, but it will be easier to deal with if you will remember this:

> While you are losing some eyesight, *you are not losing vision.*
>
> While you are losing some visual perception, *you are not losing the ability to see.*

Allow your nonvisual abilities to take over, and you will "see" the world in a whole new way. How lucky you are to have those senses in reserve and waiting for you to set them free!

Put yourself to the test by trying these simple exercises.

Make a sandwich while focusing your gaze elsewhere. Notice how easy it is to find what you need and accomplish the task if you are patient and organized.

The next time you hold your grandchild, close your eyes and let your other senses take part. There is more to that child than you ever imagined with your eyes open!

Sit outdoors with your eyes shut for ten minutes. (Try not to doze off.) Count the number of sounds, smells, and tactile sensations that identify the day. If you don't come up with at least ten, start over. You dozed off.

Close your eyes while riding in the car (as a passenger, of course) on a warm day with the window down. See if you can describe your surroundings, the direction you are traveling, and how fast you are going. Is there anything of importance that you need your eyesight for? Probably not as much as you might think.

Get ready for bed in total darkness. You will find that you need to move slowly and carefully, but you will likely discover that it's really not that difficult.

If you are successful with these kinds of exercises, you have nothing to fear from a future with visual impairment. Not only will AMD never cast you into total darkness, you will also tip the odds in your favor by introducing your other senses to their potentials.

IN A SENTENCE:

> *Seeing means more than meets the eye. You will experience seeing in many new ways if you will set all of your senses free.*

The End of the War

FOCAL POINTS:

- *Researchers are winning the war on retinal disease.*
- *You are at the battlefront.*

ALL THE research described in this book is directed at the same goal: retaining sight, the most important of all of our senses in this highly visual world. Scientists are making steady progress toward effective treatments for AMD and related retinal diseases. This offers a great deal of reason for hope—if not for your generation, certainly for your children and grandchildren.

As you read earlier, battles are being won with the help of an arsenal of treatments that are closing in from both fronts. These, however, are treatments that only help to keep the enemy at a safe distance. The war will be won when a patient can receive a diagnosis, undergo a procedure or take a few pills, and return home as a permanently fully sighted person. This section describes current research that stands a good chance of making that scenario a reality.

Gene replacement therapy

Each one of us came into this world with a whole set of inherited genes. Completed in 2003 after thirteen years of work, the massive Human Genome Project has led to a mapping of the entire genetic makeup of the human body. The best estimate so far is that there are as many as 24,500 protein-coding genes.[88] By discovering those that are related to AMD (and several have already been identified), researchers can figure out what causes them to go wrong (mutate). Because of the number of combinations of genes assigned to given tasks, that is a tedious process, but once it is accomplished, healthy genes can be delivered to retinal cells (through **viral vectors**) as replacements. These healthy genes will be better able to produce the proteins that are essential to the cell's function, allowing maintenance of normal vision.

An understanding of the genetic basis of AMD will help tremendously in the fight against the disease. With this knowledge, family members at risk can be identified through genetic testing. Scientists will then develop pharmaceutical and gene-based therapies that result in addressing the underlying genetic dysfunction that may cause AMD.

Genetic therapy, however, is but one part of the equation. You and your doctor will also need to consider behavioral, nutritional, and environmental influences, as discussed in Day 4.

Stem cell transplantation

Stem cells are undeveloped structures that are able to develop into any of the nearly 220 cell types that make up the human body and theoretically reproduce themselves ad infinitum. The discovery of adult stem cells (**progenitor cells**) in the eyes of adult rodents at the turn of the century led to promising research in the area of retinal cell transplantation.[89, 90] Stem cells, it seems, have certain characteristics of photoreceptor and retinal nerve cells, so researchers have been trying to find out if they can actually function as such. If this work is successful, stem cell transplants may be able to restore lost vision.

The most viable source of stem cells is fetal tissue. Potential sources are:

leftover, unwanted embryos from fertility clinics
donated fetuses from abortions
cloning
creating new embryos expressly for the purpose of harvesting the cells

Because of the moral issues raised over the use of embryos, alternative methods of acquiring stem cells are being sought. One possibility is harvesting them from bone marrow and brain tissue. Biologists have also discovered stem cells in umbilical cord blood and in donated human retinas.[91] All of the research on stem cells has been promising, and some nonocular diseases have already been cured as a result of it. Now the work continues in hopes of verifying the findings and determining the effectiveness of stem cell transplantation as a treatment or cure for AMD.

Artificial retina (microchip implantation)

You have probably heard of the research on artificial ("bionic") retinas. These highly experimental prosthetic devices are made of silicon computer chips. They are intended to restore ambulatory vision, giving people the freedom to walk without the assistance of a cane or guide animal.

Several research groups are working to develop an artificial retina.[92] Each group has its own variation of the science, and they report varying degrees of success. An artificial retina for AMD patients is not useful in its current design, since the amount of sight it allows is far less than the worst stage of AMD. Still, microchip research may someday lead to more refined systems for the unique needs of people with only central vision loss.

Implantable miniature telescope (IMT)

The implantable miniature microscope (IMT) is a microsized precision telescope, about the size of a pea. It is implanted in one eye of patients with significant vision loss (no better than 20/80, but not worse than 20/800 in both eyes) who are in need of cataract surgery. According to the inventors, the device has had no serious safety issues,[93] and follow-up studies have shown significant improvement in quality of life and daily living activities of those who use it. You are on the front line.

You are one of millions whose patience and courage is helping to defeat the enemy and carve out a new world of sight for every man, woman, and child from here on in. You certainly didn't ask for that awesome responsibility, but if you want to make the best of an unpleasant situation, consider volunteering for a clinical trial. Your help can really make a difference, and you might even be in the right time and place for the next breakthrough. You will also receive examinations, and maybe an effective treatment, absolutely free.

What is a clinical trial?

A clinical trial involves direct observation of a living patient to answer specific questions about vaccines, therapies, or new methods. It is designed in four phases, during which rigorous protocols must be followed under FDA guidelines:

Phase I: Determination of safety and side effects on 20–80 people

Phase II: Determination of effectiveness and safety on 200–300 people

Phase III: Confirmation of results on 1,000–3,000 people

Phase IV: Studies done after FDA approval and public use.

Testing is accomplished in "trial centers" around the country under approved clinicians, and results are carefully analyzed at each step before permission is given to move on to the next phase. Clinical trials can take years to complete and cost millions of dollars in time, professional services, product development, and equipment. Sometimes a treatment will not meet the predicted end point, which means that the trial will be stopped, either permanently or until the problem is solved to the satisfaction of the FDA.

You will have to meet certain criteria to be accepted into a trial. Such criteria are announced ahead of time, along with contact information for each testing location. In most trials, you will be randomly assigned to either an **experimental group**, which receives the actual treatment, or a **control group**, which receives a **sham** (fake) treatment. Often the design of the trial is **double-masked** (also, ironically, called **double-blind**). This means that neither you nor the researcher knows which group you are in.

Some trials are designed to determine drug dosages and side effects. No control group is used in this type of study. All subjects would receive the treatment, but in differing amounts. These are called **dose-ranging**, or **dose-escalation** trials.

You need to understand that participation in a trial does not guarantee improvement of your condition. Sometimes, the hoped-for results are not achieved. Only about one-third of experimental drugs, for example, successfully complete both Phase I and Phase II studies, and only 70 to 90 percent of drugs successfully complete Phase III testing.[94] Sometimes you might actually suffer side effects. You will be required to sign a waiver to absolve the researcher of any responsibility for this eventuality.

Clinical trials are announced and described on the Internet at www.clinicaltrials.gov and www.center-watch.com. You will also find trials announced in the print and broadcast media, and your doctor should be able to give you information about studies being conducted for your particular condition.

By becoming an active participant in a trial, you are putting yourself on the front line. Such a position may not provide the serenity of denial, but it is where you will feel in better control of your destiny. Here is a poem that expresses the pride felt by AMD people who have likewise chosen to face the challenges of visual impairment head-on.

The Promise
You came to the raging river
Where the roar gorged the air.
You cried, "Show me where you crossed over,
If you're really there."

We replied, "Yes, we're here together,
And we'll show the way to you.
But there's not yet a bridge for crossing:
Our way was not *over* but *through*."[95]

You have chosen to go *through* this process of battling AMD because there is just no easier way. You could close this book and try to ignore it, but you would find it difficult to ignore something that is literally right before you. By placing yourself at the front, however, you are facing AMD squarely and refusing to be a victim. Good for you!

IN A SENTENCE:

> You are not only witnessing the beginning of the
> end of the AMD war, you can actually have a hand
> in winning it.

MONTH **11**

Your Gift to the Future

FOCAL POINT:

▶ *You are a pioneer.*

SINCE DAY 1 of this book you have learned a great deal about AMD, not only from the experts, but from patients themselves. All of the information can be placed into one of three categories:

Causes and Symptoms
Treatments and Cures
Living Successfully

Armed with this knowledge, you have the power to squarely face the challenges of AMD. And because science is on the brink of new discoveries, you and millions of others are pioneers who will lead the world into the new age of vision. The following scene could well be about you.

CHILD: Who's in that photo, Mom?

MOM: That's my grandmother. Your *great*-grandmother.

CHILD: Can we go see her and get a present?

MOM: Not now, honey. She passed away years ago, before you born.

CHILD: Was she nice?

MOM: Very nice. She taught me how to play cards and knit and cook and all kinds of things.

CHILD: I wish I could see her.

MOM: You would think she was magic. I did.

CHILD: She was a magician?

MOM: Kind of. Grandma could tell when the bacon was done, she could tell me what I was wearing, and she could tell if I was happy or sad. All kinds of things.

CHILD: That's not magic. Anybody can do that stuff.

MOM: Without looking?

CHILD: Oh.

MOM: Remember how the doctor fixed your eyes when they got sick?

CHILD: Yeah, I got a shot.

MOM: Don't sound so grumpy. Grandma's eyes were sick, too, but her doctor didn't know how to fix her like your doctor did.

CHILD: She couldn't see?

MOM: Not very well.

CHILD: That's sad.

MOM: It could have been, but Grandma decided to help the doctors by letting them study her and try out new medicines.

CHILD: She got shots, too?

MOM: Sometimes. And the most magical thing was that Grandma was always happy.

CHILD: With all those shots? Why?

MOM: Because whenever she started to feel sad or scared, she would think of you.

CHILD: Mom, I wasn't here yet.

MOM: No, you weren't. But she knew you were coming someday; and she knew your eyes might get sick, too. Grandma helped so you wouldn't have to ever be sad or scared in that way.

CHILD: Grandma was my hero. That's a good present.

MOM: That was a *very* good present.

You can take some comfort in knowing that visual impairment will soon be something your grandchildren will only read about. The cures will come, and the next step will be restoration of vision for those who have already been affected.

In the meantime, you can help by passing along the gifts of knowledge and support to people who share your condition. You can also volunteer for clinical trials, contribute to research, or donate your eyes to science. Or you can simply set an example of courage by living your life as well as possible.

This is a time of medical miracles, and you are part of it. A wall may never bear your name. A statue may never be erected in your memory. But because you are part of this place and time, millions of people will be able to see clearly with their eyes those things you may be able to see with only your heart. You now have an opportunity to give gifts that will last forever: your knowledge, your support, and your courage. And thank you especially for your courage. That is a very good present.

learning from living

Where to Go from Here?

FOCAL POINT:

▶ *This is only the beginning of the road.*

DURING THE past six months you have gone from the practical matter of eccentric viewing training, through the many varied emotions of AMD patients, and on into a touch of philosophical thought about visual impairment. All of this set the stage for a look at the future and how you can set about preparing for it with your feet on solid ground.

When you reach the end of this final month, you will have at your fingertips as much (or more) than most AMD patients do when it comes to understanding and coping with the challenges you might have to face. No one will honestly tell you that life is easy with AMD, but most people will tell you that knowledge and support can make it almost normal. If you are willing to find alternative ways of living without visual dependence, you will be amazed at the possibilities.

This final month will lead you to organizations and practical resources, and will provide basic information about computer use—all of which will be useful to you long after you close this book. Keep it handy, as it is intended to be not only a tutorial about AMD, but a comprehensive reference as well.

Computer technology for the visually impaired

Many references have been made in this book about using the Internet to find information. If you are one of those seniors in the "lost generation" who missed out on the computer age, don't despair. It's much easier than you think!

Your first step is to get to a computer. More than 95 percent of public libraries now have computers that are freely accessible, and you might even find someone on the staff who will assist you the first time or two. Get there early in the day, however, and avoid Saturdays. Otherwise, you may have to wait in line.

If you live in a retirement center or assisted living facility, there may be a computer room already set up for you. Most larger centers provide this service, along with a person who can help. If there is no such person on hand, make friends with another resident who knows what they are doing. Most people are very happy to pass along what they have learned.

Your own computer

Maybe you would rather have your own private computer. You can pick up a good laptop model now for less than eight hundred dollars (and many desktop models are even cheaper), and for an additional investment, classes for seniors can usually be found at libraries, churches, and community colleges. Call around. There will also be a monthly fee of between ten and thirty dollars for subscribing to Internet access through a company (called an Internet service provider) such as AOL, Earthlink, Juno, and SBC Global, just to name a few of many choices. You will also need to connect your computer to either a phone line or to a special cable installed in your home or apartment. Telephone companies like Sprint, AT&T, SBC, and Verizon offer "digital subscriber lines" (DSL) for high-speed connection to the Internet. These companies also offer "wireless Internet" (also known as "wireless Web" or "mobile Web") for people who want to surf the Internet using cell phones. Less expensive, but slower, is "dial-up" access, which uses a traditional phone line.

Special software

If your vision is such that you cannot read a computer monitor (and there's nothing wrong with putting your nose on it to do so), learn how to use screen magnification software. Software refers to programs that are transferred to a computer's hard drive ("installed") from a disc or from a file downloaded from the Internet. Basic magnification software may be built in to the computer, or it may have to be purchased separately and installed. You can also adjust the monitor's brightness and contrast to suit your needs.

In the event that you acquire your own computer and need more magnification than it provides, you can purchase and install software such as BigShot, Home Page Reader, Web Eyes, and ZoomText. If even strong magnification doesn't help, some computers come with screen readers installed that will read the text aloud from your monitor. You can also purchase screen reader software separately under such brand names as Jaws, Open Book, OutSpoken, TextAloud, Text Reader, Text-to-Audio, and Universal Reader.

As if that isn't enough help, you don't even need to type. You can simply speak into a microphone, and your computer can do the typing for you. With this technology, you can use voice commands to operate your computer, and you can even write e-mail messages without touching your keypad. Such software comes under names like CaptionMic, CART, C-Print, Dragon Naturally Speaking, RapidText, and TypeWell.

And finally, a product called Freedom Box allows you to navigate the Internet, send e-mail, and participate in "chat rooms" totally by voice or key commands, all without a traditional computer and monitor setup. Basically, you speak to the "box" (which looks like a keypad), telling it where you want to go on the Internet. It connects you, and then it reads the information for you when you get there. A monthly subscription fee is charged for the service and Internet connection.

You will find that the cost of such software will vary greatly, depending upon the capabilities of the programs. Your best approach is to contact a low vision therapist who can work with you on finding just the right program for your needs. If you decide, however, to shop on your own, take advantage of free trial offers, which are normally good for thirty days. If no free trial is available, be sure the product has a money-back guarantee. Most of the products mentioned here can be obtained through the dealers listed in Appendix C.

Macular degeneration organizations

More than a dozen nonprofit organizations in the United States offer information and support to AMD patients. Below is a *nonselective* directory of all such organizations. Also included are two umbrella organizations that represent a large number of additional groups worldwide.

Inclusion in this list is not necessarily an endorsement. The effectiveness of a service organization is best defined by its *activities, accomplishments,* and *financial management.* Opinions about the effectiveness of an organization should, therefore, be based upon subjective criteria such as:

Satisfaction of all statements made in the organization's publicized description.

Appropriate use of public contributions and grants. Financial information is available online from GuideStar: The Donor's Guide to the Charitable Universe (www.guidestar.org).

Proof of honesty in advertising, full disclosure, and other accepted principles of conduct. Certification of Web sites is available from the Center for Applied Special Technology (www.cast.org).

Web site meets minimum standards for low vision access. Certification is available from the Health on the Net Foundation(www.hon.ch).

Solicitation methods meet acceptable ethical standards.

You are encouraged to consider all of these criteria before patronizing or contributing to these or any other charitable groups.

AMD Alliance International
1929 Bayview Avenue
Toronto, Ontario M4G 3E8
Canada
Telephone: (416) 486-2500, ext. 7505
Web site: www.amdalliance.org

American Macular Degeneration Foundation
PO Box 515
Northampton, MA 01061-0515
Telephone: (413) 268-7660
Web site: www.macular.org

Association for Macular Diseases
Manhattan Eye, Ear and Throat Hospital, 8th floor
210 E. 64th Street
New York, NY 10021
Telephone: (212) 605-3719
Web site: www.macula.org

The Foundation Fighting Blindness
11435 Cronhill Drive
Owings Mills, MD 21117-2220
Telephone: (888) 394-3937
Web site: www.blindness.org

The Macula Foundation
Manhattan Eye, Ear and Throat Hospital, 8th floor
210 E. 64th Street
New York, NY 10021
Telephone: (212) 605-3777
Web site: www.macula.org/foundation

Macula Vision Research Foundation
Five Tower Bridge
300 Barr Harbor Drive, Suite 600
West Conshohocken, PA 19428
Telephone: (610) 668-6705
Web site: www.mvrf.org

Macular Degeneration Foundation
PO Box 531313
Henderson, NV 89053
Telephone: (888) 633-3937
Web site: www.eyesight.org

Macular Degeneration International
6700 N. Oracle Road, Suite 505
Tucson, AZ 85704-7733
Telephone: (800) 683-5555
Web site: www.maculardegeneration.org

Macular Degeneration Partnership
The Discovery Fund for Eye Research
8733 Beverly Boulevard, Suite 201
Los Angeles, CA 90048
Telephone: (888) 430-9898
Web site: www.amd.org

Macular Degeneration Research
American Health Assistance Foundation
22512 Gateway Center Drive
Clarksburg, MD 20871
Telephone: (800) 437-2423
Web site: www.ahaf.org

Macular Degeneration Support
3600 Blue Ridge
Grandview, MO 64030-1561
Telephone: (816) 761-7080
Web site: www.mdsupport.org

Macular Disease Society
Darwin House
13a Bridge Street
Andover, Hampshire SP10 1BE
United Kingdom
Telephone: 011 44 1264 350 551
Web site: www.maculardisease.org

Prevent Blindness America
211 W. Wacker Drive, Suite 1700
Chicago, IL 60606
Telephone: (800) 331-2020
Web site: www.preventblindness.org

Research to Prevent Blindness
645 Madison Avenue
New York, NY 10022-1010
Telephone: (800) 621-0026
Web site: www.rpbusa.org

Further reading

If this book has only whetted your appetite, here is further recommended reading for you.

Age-Related Macular Degeneration, Jeffrey W. Berger (ed.), Stuart L. Fine, Maureen G. Maguire (St. Louis, MO: Mosby, 1999).

Bert's Eye View: Coping with Macular Degeneration, Bertram Silverman and Nina Fuller (Portland, ME: Viewpoint, 1997).

Coping with Low Vision (Coping with Aging Series), Marshall E. Flax, Bette L. McCaulley, Don J. Golembiewski (San Diego: Singular Publishing Group, 1993).

Coping with Macular Degeneration: Sound, Helpful Information for Those Who Must Deal with This Degenerative Vision Disorder, Linda Comac, Ira Marc Price (New York: Avery, 1999).

The Lighthouse Handbook on Vision Impairment and Vision Rehabilitation, Barbara Silverstone, et al. (eds.) (New York: Oxford University Press, 2000).

Living with Vision Loss: Independence, Driving, and Low Vision Solutions, Daniel Gottlieb, Cheryl H. Allen, Jane Eikenberry, Susan Ingall-Woodruff, and Marianne Johnson (Decatur, GA: Saint Barthélemy Press, 1998).

Macular Degeneration: The Latest Scientific Discoveries and Treatments for Preserving Your Sight, Robert D'Amato, MD, Joan Snyder, MD (New York: Walker, 2000).

Macular Degeneration: Living Positively with Vision Loss, Betty Wason with James J. McMillan, MD (Alameda, CA: Hunter House, 1998).

Macular Degeneration: The Complete Guide to Saving and Maximizing Your Sight—2nd edition (Large print), Lylas G. Mogk, MD, and Marja Mogk, PhD (New York: Ballantine, 2003).

Out of the Corner of My Eye: Living with Vision Loss in Later Life (Large print), Nicolette Pernot Ringgold (New York: American Foundation for the Blind, 1991). Also available on cassette.

Overcoming Macular Degeneration: A Guide to Seeing Beyond the Clouds, Yale Solomon, MD, and Jonathan D. Solomon (New York: HarperCollins/ Wholecare, 2000).

Twilight: Losing Sight, Gaining Insight, Henry A. Grunwald (New York: Knopf, 1999).

As you see, a huge system of support and information is at your disposal. You have more knowledge and human interconnection than anyone has ever had before, so you are truly not alone. Make a phone call, turn a page, or tap some keys on a computer, and a world of help is available to you, all due to the hard work of thousands of people who understand exactly what you need to maximize your vision and the quality of your life.

Keep this book on hand for looking up information when you need it. Reread the personal accounts of the very real people contained in its pages. And most important of all, think often of the future generations who will see the world clearer and brighter because you were here.

Appendix A

DIRECTORY OF AGENCIES FOR
THE VISUALLY IMPAIRED

Alabama

Alabama Council of the Blind
Telephone: (800) 424-8666
Web site: www.acb-alabama.org

Alabama Department of Rehabilitation Blind Services
2129 E. South Boulevard
PO Box 11586
Montgomery, AL 36111-0586
Telephone: (334) 281-8780
Web site: www.rehab.state.al.us

Alabama Vocational Rehabilitation Services
Lakeshore Rehabilitation Facility
PO Box 591273830 Ridgeway Drive
Birmingham, AL 35259-9127
Telephone: (205) 870-5999 or (800) 441-7609
Web site: www.jan.wvu.edu/SBSES/VOCREHAB.HTM

National Federation of the Blind of Alabama
3339 S. Perry Street
Montgomery, AL 36105
Telephone: (205) 264-7547
Web site: www.nfbofalabama.org

Alaska

Alaska Division of Vocational Rehabilitation
Visual Impairment or Blindness
801 W. Tenth Street, Suite A
Juneau, AK 99801-1894
Telephone: (907) 465-2814 or (800) 478-2815
Web site: www.labor.state.ak.us/dvr/home.htm

Arizona

Arizona Council of the Blind
Telephone: (800) 424-8666
Web site: www.acb.org/arizona/fsmarjd.html

Arizona Center for the Blind and Visually Impaired
3100 E. Roosevelt Street
Phoenix, AZ 7411
Telephone: (602) 273-7411
Web site: www.acbvi.org

Arizona Services for Rehabilitation and Visually Impaired
1789 W. Jefferson, 2nd Floor NW, 930-A
Phoenix, AZ 85007
Telephone: (602) 542-6289
Web site: www.de.state.az.us/rsa/blind.asp

National Federation of the Blind of Arizona
311 W. McNair Street
Chandler, AZ 85224
Telephone: (602) 892-4387 or (602) 892-4387
Web site: www.nfbarizona.com

Arkansas

American Council of the Blind of Arkansas
Telephone: (800) 424-8666
Web site: www.acb.org/affiliates

Arkansas Division of Services for the Blind
522 Main Street, Suite 100
Little Rock, AR 72201
Telephone: (501) 682-5463 or (800) 960-9270
Web site: www.arkansas.gov/dhhs/dsb/NEWDSB/index.htm

Arkansas Division of Vocational Rehabilitation
1616 Brookwood Drive
Little Rock, AR 72203
Telephone: (501) 296-1661
Web site: www.arsinfo.org

National Federation of the Blind of Arkansas
19 Brooklawn Drive
Little Rock, AR 72205-2304
Telephone: (501) 228-9751
Web site: www.geocities.com/SouthBeach/Pointe/3226

California

American Council of the Blind of California
Telephone: (800) 424-8666
Web site: www.acb.org/affiliates

American Foundation for the Blind–West
111 Pine Street, Suite 725
San Francisco, CA 94111
Telephone: (415) 392-4845
Web site: www.afb.org

California Department of Rehabilitation Services
PO Box 944222
Sacramento, CA 94244-2220
Telephone: (916) 263-8981
Web site: www.dss.cahwnet.gov/cdssweb/blindservi_187.htm

National Federation of the Blind of California
175 E. Olive Avenue, Suite 308
Burbank, CA 91502-1812
Telephone: (818) 558-6524
Web site: www.nfbcal.org

Colorado

American Council of the Blind of Colorado
1536 Wynkoop Street, Suite 203
Denver, CO 80202
Telephone: (303) 831-0117 or (888) 775-2221
Web site: www.acbco.org

Colorado Division of Rehabilitation Services
Red Rock Park Office Building
207 Canyon Boulevard, Suite 202
Boulder, CO 80301
Telephone: (303) 444-2816
Web site: http://bcn.boulder.co.us/human-social/center.html

National Federation of the Blind of Colorado
1660 S. Albion Street, Suite 918
Denver, CO 80222
Telephone: (303) 504-5979
Web site: www.nfbco.org

Connecticut

American Council of the Blind of Connecticut
191 Center Brooke Road
Hamden, CT 06518
Telephone: (800) 231-3349
Web site: www.acb.org/affiliates

Connecticut Board of Education and Services for the Blind
184 Windsor Avenue
Windsor, CT 06095
Telephone: (860) 602-4000
Web site: www.besb.state.ct.us

Connecticut Rehabilitation Services
Board of Education and Services for the Blind
170 Ridge Road
Wethersfield, CT 06109
Telephone: (860) 566-5800
Web site: www.ct.gov/dss/site/default.asp

National Federation of the Blind of Connecticut
580 Burnside Avenue, Suite#1
East Hartford, CT 06108
Telephone: (860) 289-1971
Web site: www.nfbct.org

Delaware

American Council of the Blind of Delaware
Telephone: (800) 424-8666
Web site: www.dcbvi.org

Delaware Division for the Visually Impaired
Delaware Department of Health and Social Services
Herman Holloway Campus
Biggs Building
1901 N. DuPont Highway
New Castle, DE 19720-1199
Telephone: (302) 577-4731
Web site: www.dhss.delaware.gov/dhss/dvi/index.html

Delaware Division of Vocational Rehabilitation
4425 N. Market Street
PO Box 9969
Wilmington, DE 19809-0969
Telephone: (302) 761-8275
Web site: www.state.de.us/deptlabor/dvr/welcome.shtml

National Federation of the Blind of Delaware
244 Green Blade Drive
Dover, DE 19904-2646
Telephone: (302) 734-1491
Web site: www.nfb.org/localorg.htm

District of Columbia

American Council of the Blind of DC
Telephone: (800) 424-8666
Web site: www.acb.org/affiliates

District of Columbia Rehabilitation Services
Department of Human Services
441 Fourth Street, NW
Washington, DC 20001
Telephone: (202) 727-1000
Web site: www.disabilityresources.org/DC.html

National Federation of the Blind of the District of Columbia
627 Dahlia Street
Washington, DC 20012
Telephone: (202) 882-8090
Web site: www.nfb.org/localorg.htm

Florida

American Council of the Blind of Florida
Telephone: (800) 424-8666
Web site: www.fcb.org

Florida Division of Blind Services
Rehabilitation Center for the Blind
1111 Willis Avenue
Daytona Beach, FL 32114
Telephone: (904) 258-4444 or (800) 741-3826
Web site: http://dbs.myflorida.com

Florida Division of Vocational Rehabilitation
Building A
2002 Old St. Augustine Road
Tallahassee, FL 32399-0696
Telephone: (850) 488-6210
Web site: www2.myflorida.com

National Federation of the Blind of Florida
121 Deer Lake Circle
Ormond Beach, FL 32174-4266
Telephone: (888) 282-5972 (preferred #) or (386) 677-6886
Web site: www.nfbflorida.org

Georgia

American Council of the Blind of Georgia
Telephone: (800) 424-8666
Web site: www.georgiacounciloftheblind.org

American Foundation for the Blind–Southeast
100 Peachtree Street, Suite 620
Atlanta, GA 30303
Telephone: (404) 525-2303
Web site: www.afb.org

Georgia Division of Services for the Blind and Visually Impaired
2 Peachtree Street NW, Suite 35-412
Atlanta, GA 30303-3166
Telephone: (404) 657-3005
Web site: www.vocrehabga.org

National Federation of the Blind of Georgia
3020 Rollingwood Lane SE
Atlanta, GA 30316-4428
Telephone: (404) 212-2021
Web site: www.nfb.org/localorg.htm

Hawaii

Hawaii Association of the Blind
Telephone: (800) 424-8666
Web site: www.acb.org/hawaii

National Federation of the Blind
PO Box 4482
Honolulu, HI 96812-4482
Telephone: (808) 391-1214
Web site: http://hi.nfbweb.org

Vocational Rehabilitation and Services for the Blind
Department of Human Services
1000 Bishop Street, Room 615
Honolulu, HI 96813
Telephone: (808) 586-5366
Web site: www.state.hi.us/dhs

Idaho

American Council of the Blind of Idaho
Telephone: (800) 424-8666
Web site: www.acb.org/affiliates

Idaho Commission for the Blind and Visually Impaired
341 W. Washington
Boise, ID 83702
Telephone: (208) 334-3220
Web site: http://adm.idaho.gov

Idaho Division of Rehabilitation Services
PO Box 83720
650 W. State Street, Room 150
Boise, ID 83720-0096
Telephone: (208) 334-3390
Web site: www.vr.idaho.gov

National Federation of the Blind of Idaho
1301 S. Capitol Boulevard
Boise, ID, 83706-2926
Telephone: (208) 343-1377
Web site: www.nfbidaho.org

Illinois

American Council of the Blind of Illinois
Telephone: (800) 424-8666
Web site: www.icbonline.org

American Foundation for the Blind–Midwest
401 N. Michigan Avenue, Suite 308
Chicago, IL 60611
Telephone: (312) 245-9961
Web site: www.afb.org

Illinois Division of Rehabilitation Services for the Blind
Bureau of Blind Services
623 E. Adams
PO Box 19429
Springfield, IL 62794-9429
Telephone: (217) 782-2093 or (800) 275-3677
Web site: www.dhs.state.il.us

Jesse Brown VA Medical Center
Visual Impairment Center to Optimize Remaining Sight (VICTORS)
820 South Damen Avenue
Chicago, IL 60612
Telephone: (312) 569-8387
Web site: www.va.gov

National Federation of the Blind of Illinois
3527 12th Avenue
Moline, IL 61265-3402
Telephone: (309) 762-NFBI (6324)
Web site: www.nfbofillinois.org/index.html

Indiana

American Council of the Blind of Indiana
Telephone: (800) 424-8666
Web site: www.acb.org/indiana

Indiana Family and Social Services Administration
Blind and Visually Impaired Services
Indiana Government Center
402 W. Washington Street, Room W453
PO Box 7083
Indianapolis, IN 46207-7083
Telephone: (317) 232-1433
Web site: www.in.gov/fssa

Indiana Vocational Rehabilitation Services
302 W. Second Street
Bloomington, IN 47403
Telephone: (812) 332-7331 or TDD (812) 332-9372
Web site: www.in.gov/fssa/servicedisabl/vr/index.html

National Federation of the Blind of Indiana
6010 Winn Penny Lane
Indianapolis, IN 46220-5253
Telephone: (317) 205-9226
Web site: www.nfb.org/localorg.htm

Iowa

Iowa Council of the United Blind
Telephone: (800) 424-8666
Web site: www.acb.org/iowa

Iowa State Department for the Blind
524 Fourth Street
Des Moines, IA 50309-2364
Telephone: (515) 281-1333 or (800) 362-2587
Web site: www.blind.state.ia.us

Iowa Division of Vocational Rehabilitation Services
510 E. 12th Street
Des Moines, IA 50319
Telephone: (515) 281-4311
Web site: www.dvrs.state.ia.us

National Federation of the Blind of Iowa
805 Fifth Avenue
Grinnell, IA 50112-1653
Telephone: (641) 236-3366
Web site: www.nfbi.org

Kansas

Kansas Association of the Blind and Visually Impaired
603 SW Topeka Blvd., Suite 303
Topeka, KS 66612
Telephone: (800) 799-1499 or (785) 235-8990
Web site: www.kabvi.org

Kansas Department of Social and Rehabilitation Services
915 SW Harrison Street
Topeka, KS 66612
Telephone: (785) 296-3959
Web site: www.srskansas.org

Kansas Division of Vocational Rehabilitation Services
Division of Services for the Blind
300 SW Oakley
Topeka, KS 66606
Telephone: (913) 296-4454
Web site: www.srskansas.org/rehab/text/VR.htm

National Federation of the Blind of Kansas
11905 Mohawk Lane
Shawnee Mission, KS 66209
Telephone: (913) 339-9341
Web site: www.nfbks.org

Kentucky

Kentucky Council of the Blind
148 Vernon Avenue
Louisville, KY 40206
Telephone: (800) 424-8666 or (502) 895-4598
Web site: www.kentucky-acb.org

Kentucky Office for the Blind
PO Box 757
209 St. Clair Street
Frankfort, KY 40602-0757
Telephone: (800) 321-6668 or (502) 564-4754
Web site: http://blind.ky.gov

Kentucky Division of Vocational Rehabilitation Services
209 St. Clair Street
Frankfort KY 40601
Telephone: (502) 564-4440 or (800) 372-7172
Web site: kydvr.state.ky.us

National Federation of the Blind of Kentucky
210 Cambridge Drive
Louisville, KY 40214-2809
Telephone: (502) 366-2317
Web site: www.nfbky.org/index.htm

Louisiana

American Council of the Blind of Louisiana
Telephone: (800) 424-8666
Web site: www.acb.org/affiliates

Louisiana Center for the Blind
101 S. Trenton
Ruston, LA 71270
Telephone: (318) 251-2891 or (800) 234-4166
Web site: www.lcb-ruston.com

Louisiana State Division of Blind Services
Department of Rehabilitation
8225 Florida Boulevard
Baton Rouge, LA 70806-4834
Telephone: (225) 925-4131; (225) 925-3594
Web site: www.dss.state.la.us/departments/lrs/Blind_Services.html

Louisiana Division of Vocational Rehabilitation Services
A. Z. Young Building
755 Third Street
Baton Rouge, LA 70802
Telephone: (225) 342-0286
Web site: www.dss.state.la.us

National Federation of the Blind of Louisiana
605 University Boulevard
Ruston, LA 71270-4862
Telephone: (318) 251-1511
Web site: www.nfbla.org/index.htm

Maine

American Council of the Blind of Maine
Telephone: (800) 424-8666
Web site: www.acb.org/affiliates

Maine Division of Services for the Blind and Visually Impaired
Maine Department of Labor
35 Anthony Avenue
State House Station Number 150
Augusta, ME 04333-0150
Telephone: (207) 624-5323
Web site: www.maine.gov/rehab

Maine Department of Special Education Services
23 State House Station
Augusta, ME 04333-0023
Telephone: (207) 287-5950
Web site: www.maine.gov/education/speced/specserv.htm

Maine Rehabilitation Center for the Blind and Visually Impaired
189 Park Avenue
Portland, ME 04102
Telephone: (207) 774-6273 or (800) 715-0097
Web site: www.maine.gov/rehab

National Federation of the Blind of Maine
88 Shaker Road
Gray, ME 04039-9707
Telephone: (207) 657-2829
Web site: www.nfb.org/localorg.htm

Maryland

American Council of the Blind of Maryland
Telephone: (800) 424-8666
Web site: www.acb-md.org

Blind Industries and Services of Maryland
2901 Strickland Street
Baltimore, MD 21223
Telephone: (410) 233-4567
Web site: www.bism.com

Maryland Division of Rehabilitation Services
1515 W. Mount Royal Avenue
Baltimore, MD 21217-4247
Telephone: (410) 333-6119
Web site: www.dpscs.state.md.us/rehabservs

Maryland Divison of Rehabilitation Services
Office for Blindness and Vision Services
2301 Argonne Drive
Baltimore, MD 21218
Telephone: (410) 554-9277 or (866) 614-4780
Web site: www.dors.state.md.us

National Federation of the Blind of Maryland
9013 Nelson Way
Columbia, MD 21045-5148
Telephone: (410) 715-9596
Web site: www.nfb.org/localorg.htm

Massachusetts

Bay State Council of the Blind
Telephone: (800) 424-8666
Web site: www.acb.org/baystate

Foundation Fighting Blindness
Massachusetts Affiliate
PO Box 850139
Braintree, MA 02185
Telephone: (781) 284-1466
Web site: www.ffb.org

Lowell Association for the Blind
174 Central Street
Lowell, MA 01852
Telephone: (978) 454-5704
Web site: www.lowellassociationfortheblind.org

Massachusetts Association for the Blind
200 Ivy Street
Brookline, MA 02446
Telephone: (800) 682-9200
Web site: www.mablind.org

Massachusetts Commission for the Blind
88 Kingston Street
Boston, MA 02111
Telephone: (617) 727-5550 or (800) 392-6450
Web site: www.mass.gov

Massachusetts Division of Vocational Rehabilitation
Administrative Offices
Fort Point Place
27-43 Wormwood Street
Boston, MA 02210-1616
Telephone: (Voice or TDD) (800) 245-6543 or (617) 204-3600
Web site: www.mass.gov

National Federation of the Blind of Massachusetts
140 Wood Street
Somerset, MA 02726
Telephone: (508) 679-8543
Web site: www.nfbmass.org

Michigan

American Council of the Blind of Michigan
Telephone: (800) 424-8666
Web site: www.acb.org/affiliates

Greater Detroit Agency for the Blind and Visually Impaired
16625 Grand River Avenue
Detroit, MI 48227
Telephone: (313) 272-3900
Web site: www.gdabvi.org

Michigan Association for the Blind and Visually Impaired
215 Sheldon SE
Grand Rapids, MI 49503
Telephone: (616) 458-1187 or (800) 466-8084
Web site: www.abvimichigan.org

Michigan Rehabilitation Services
Victor Office Center, 1st Floor
201 N. Washington Square
Lansing, MI 48913
Telephone: (517) 241-4000 or (888) 605-6722
Web site: www.michigan.gov

National Federation of the Blind of Michigan
1212 N. Foster Avenue
Lansing, MI 48912-3309
Telephone: (517) 372-8700
Web site: www.nfbmi.org

Minnesota

American Council of the Blind of Minnesota
Telephone: (800) 424-8666
Web site: www.acb.org/minnesota

Minnesota Division of Vocational Rehabilitation Services
390 N. Robert Street
St. Paul, MN 55101
Telephone: (651) 296-5616 or (800) 328-9095; TTY (651) 296-3900
Web site: www.deed.state.mn.us/rehab/vr/main_vr.htm

Minnesota State Services for the Blind
390 N. Robert Street
St. Paul, MN 55101
Telephone: (651) 284-3300 or (800) 652-9000
Web site: www.mnssb.org

National Federation of the Blind of Minnesota
100 East 22nd Street
Minneapolis, MN 55404
Telephone: (612) 872-9363
Web site: http://members.tcq.net/nfbmn

Mississippi

American Council of the Blind of Mississippi
Telephone: (800) 424-8666
Web site: www.acb.org/mcb

Mississippi Department of Rehabilitation Services for the Blind
PO Box 1698
Jackson, MS 39215-1698
Telephone: (601) 853-5100 or (800) 443-1000
Web site: www.mdrs.state.ms.us

National Federation of the Blind of Mississippi
268 Lexington Avenue
Jackson, MS 39209
Telephone: (601) 969-3352
Web site: www.nfb.org/localorg.htm

Missouri

American Council of the Blind of Missouri
Telephone: (800) 424-8666
Web site: www.acb.org/missouri

Kansas City VA Medical Center
Visual Impairment Center to Optimize Remaining Sight (VICTORS)
4801 Linwood Boulevard
Kansas City, MO 64128
Telephone: (816) 861-4700
Web site: www.va.gov

Missouri Division of Vocational Rehabilitation Services
3024 W. Truman Boulevard
Jefferson City, MO 65109
Telephone: (573) 526-7004 or toll-free (877) 222-8963
Web site: www.dss.mo.gov/fsd/rsb/vr.htmv

Missouri Rehabilitation Services for the Blind
615 E. 13th Street, Room 409
Kansas City, MO 64106
Telephone: (816) 889-2677
Web site: www.dss.mo.gov/fsd/rsb

National Federation of the Blind of Missouri
3910 Tropical Lane
Columbia, MO 65202-6205
Telephone: (573) 874-1774
Web site: www.nfbmo.org

Montana

National Federation of the Blind of Montana
408 W. Sussex Avenue
Missoula, MT 59801
Telephone: (406) 549-1868
Web site: www.nfb.org/localorg.htm

Nebraska

American Council of the Blind of Nebraska
Telephone: (800) 424-8666
Web site: www.acb.org/nebraska

Nebraska Department of Services for the Visually Impaired
4600 Valley Road, Suite 100
Lincoln, NE 68510
Telephone: (402) 471-8100
Web site: www.hhs.state.ne.us

Nebraska Division of Vocational Rehabilitation
PO Box 94987
301 Centennial Mall South
Lincoln, NE 68509-4987
Telephone: (402) 471-3644
Web site: www.vocrehab.state.ne.us

National Federation of the Blind of Nebraska
6210 Walker Avenue
Lincoln, NE 68507-2468
Telephone: (402) 465-5468
Web site: nfbn.inebraska.com

Nevada

National Federation of the Blind of Nevada
1401 N. Michael Way
Unit 118 L
Las Vegas, NV 89108
Telephone: (702) 639-9072
Web site: www.nfb.org/localorg.htm

Nevada Council of the Blind
Telephone: (800) 424-8666
Web site: www.acb.org/nevada

Nevada Division of Vocational Rehabilitation Services
505 E. King Street, Room 502
Carson City, NV 89701-3705
Telephone: (702) 687-4440
Web site: http://detr.state.nv.us

Nevada Services for the Blind and Visually Impaired
505 E. King Street, Room 505
Carson City, NV 89701
Telephone: (702) 687-4440
Web site: http://detr.state.nv.us/rehab/reh_bvi.htm

New Hampshire

New Hampshire Division of Services for the Blind and Visually Impaired
78 Regional Drive, Building 2
Concord, NH 03301-8508
Telephone: (603) 271-3537
Web site: www.nfb.org/localorg.htm

New Hampshire Vocational Rehabilitation Services
78 Regional Drive
Concord, NH 03301
Telephone: (603) 271-3471 or (800) 299-1647
Web site: www.ed.state.nh.us

National Federation of the Blind of New Hampshire
40 Chestnut Street, Apt. 604
Dover, NH 03820
Telephone: (603) 524-1945
Web site: www.nfb.org/states/entry/nh.htm

New Jersey

National Federation of the Blind of New Jersey
254 Spruce Street
Bloomfield, NJ 07003
Telephone: (866) 632-1940 or (973) 743-0075
Web site: www.nfb.org/localorg.htm

New Jersey Commission for the Blind and Visually Impaired
PO Box 4701
7153 Halsey Street
Newark, NJ 07101
Telephone: (973) 648-2324
Web site: www.state.nj.us/humanservices/cbvi/index.html

New Jersey Council of the Blind
Telephone: (800) 424-8666
Web site: www.acb.org/affiliates/index.html

New Jersey Division of Services for Vocational Rehabilitation
135 E. State Street
PO Box 398
Trenton, NJ 08625-0398
Telephone: (609) 292-5987
Web site: www.nj.gov/labor/dvrs/vrsindex.html

New Jersey Foundation for the Blind
230 Diamond Spring Road
Danville, NJ 07834
Telephone: (973) 627-0055
www.njffb.org

New Mexico

American Council of the Blind of New Mexico
Telephone: (800) 424-8666
Web site: www.acb.org/affiliates

Las Luminarias of the New Mexico Council of the Blind
2119 Broadway Boulevard SE
Albuquerque, NM 87102-4954
Telephone: (505) 247-0441

National Federation of the Blind of New Mexico
1331 Park Avenue SW, Suite 1504
Albuquerque, NM 87102
Telephone: (505) 243-6165
Web site: www.nfbnm.org

New Mexico Commission for the Blind
2905 Rodeo Park Drive East, Bldg. 4, Suite 100
Santa Fe, NM 87505
Telephone: (505) 476-4479 or toll-free (888) 513-7968
Web site: www.state.nm.us/cftb/Introduction.html

New Mexico Division of Vocational Rehabilitation Services
435 St. Michael's Drive, Building D
Santa Fe, NM 87505
Telephone: (505) 476-4479 or toll-free (888) 513-7968
Web site: www.state.nm.us/cftb/VocationalRehabilitation.html

New Mexico State Commission for the Blind
Administrative Office
P.E.R.A. Building, Room 553
Santa Fe, NM 87503
Telephone: (505) 827-4479 or (888) 513-7968
Web site: www.state.nm.us/cftb

New York

American Council of the Blind of New York
Telephone: (800) 424-8666
Web site: www.acbny.org

American Foundation for the Blind
11 Penn Plaza, Suite 300
New York, NY 10001
Telephone: (212) 502-7600
Web site: www.afb.org

National Federation of the Blind of New York
471 63rd Street
Brooklyn, NY 11220-4617
Telephone: (718) 567-7821
Web site: www.nfbny.org

Northport VA Medical Center
Visual Impairment Center to Optimize Remaining Sight (VICTORS)
79 Middleville Road
Northport, NY 11768
Telephone: (631) 261-4400
Web site: www.va.gov

New York Division of Services for the Blind and Visually Impaired
Visions
500 Greenwich Street, 3rd Floor
New York, NY 10013-1354
Telephone: (212) 625-1616 / Fax: (212) 219-4078
Web site: www.visionsvcb.org

New York State Commission for the Blind and Visually Impaired
Department of Social Services
40 N. Pearl Street
Albany, NY 12243
Telephone: (518) 473-1801 or (866) 871-3000
Web site: www.ocfs.state.ny.us/main/cbvh

New York Vocational and Educational Services for Individuals with Disabilities (VESID)
One Commerce Plaza, Room 1624
Albany, NY 12234
Telephone: (800) 222-5627
Web site: www.vesid.nysed.gov

Northeastern Association for the Blind in Albany
301 Washington Avenue
Albany, NY 12206
Telephone: (518) 463-1211
Web site: www.naba-vision.org

North Carolina

American Council of the Blind of North Carolina
Telephone: (800) 424-8666
Web site: www.nccounciloftheblind.org

National Federation of the Blind of North Carolina
128 Summerlea Drive
Charlotte, NC 28214-1324
Telephone: (704) 391-3204
Web site: www.nfbofnc.org

North Carolina Division of Services for the Blind
309 Ashe Avenue
Raleigh, NC 27606
Telephone: (919) 733-9822
Web site: www.dhhs.state.nc.us/dsb

North Carolina Division of Vocational Rehabilitation
2001 Mail Service Center
Adams Building, 101 Blair Drive
Raleigh, NC 27699-2001
Telephone: (919) 733-3364
Web site: www.dhhs.state.nc.us/docs/divinfo/dvr.htm

North Dakota

North Dakota Association of the Blind
2542 17th Street North East
Manvel, ND 58256
Telephone: (701) 696-2509
Web site: www.ndab.org

National Federation of the Blind of North Dakota
111 18th Street South, Apartment 4
Fargo, ND 58103
Telephone: (218) 790-2899
Web site: www.nfb.org/localorg.htm

North Dakota Division of Rehabilitation Services
600 S. Second Street, Suite 1B
Bismarck, ND 58504-5729
Telephone: (701) 328-8950
Web site: www.nd.gov/humanservices/services/disabilities

North Dakota Vision Services/School for the Blind (NDVS)
500 Stanford Road, Suite A
Grand Forks, ND 58203-2799
Telephone: (701) 795-2700
Web site: www.ndvisionservices.com

Ohio

American Council of the Blind of Ohio
Telephone: (800) 424-8666
Web site: www.acbohio.org

National Federation of the Blind of Ohio
237 Oak Street
Oberlin, OH 44074
Telephone: (216) 775-2216
Web site: www.nfbohio.org

Ohio Division of Services for the Visually Impaired
Rehabilitation Services Commission
400 E. Campus View Boulevard
Columbus, OH 43235-4604
Telephone: (614) 438-1255
Web site: www.rsc.ohio.gov/VR_Services/BSVI/bsvi.asp

Ohio Division of Vocational Rehabilitation Services
400 E. Campus View Boulevard
Columbus, OH 43235-4604
Telephone: (800) 282-4536
Web site: www.rsc.ohio.gov/VR_Services/BVR/bvr.html

Oklahoma

American Council of the Blind of Oklahoma
Telephone: (800) 424-8666
Web site: www.okcb.org

National Federation of the Blind of Oklahoma
13258 E. 29th Place
Tulsa, OK 74134
Telephone: (918) 641-0700
Web site: www.nfb.org/localorg.htm

Oklahoma Department of Rehabilitation Services
Visual Services Division
3535 NW 58th Street, Suite 500
Oklahoma City, OK 73112-4815
Telephone: (405) 951-3400
Web site: www.okrehab.org

Oregon

American Council of the Blind of Oregon
Telephone: (800) 424-8666
Web site: www.acboforegon.org

National Federation of the Blind of Oregon
5005 Main Street
Springfield, OR 97478-6065
Telephone: (541) 726-6924
Web site: www.nfb-or.org

Oregon Commission for the Blind
535 SE 12th Avenue
Portland, OR 97214
Telephone: (971) 673-1588 or toll-free (888) 202-5463
Web site: www.oregon.gov/Blind/index.shtml

Oregon Division of Vocational Rehabilitation Services
1400 Queen Avenue SE, Suite 107
Albany, OR 97321
Telephone: (541) 967-2022
Web site: www.rsc.ohio.gov/VR_Services/BVR/bvr.html

Oregon Department of Human Services
500 Summer Street NE
Salem, OR 97310-1098
Telephone: (503) 945-5811 or (800) 282-8096
Web site: www.dhs.state.or.us/disabilities

Pennsylvania

Associated Services for the Blind of the Delaware Valley
919 Walnut Street, 5th Floor
Philadelphia, PA 19107
Telephone: (215) 627-0600
Web site: www.asb.org

Golden Triangle Council of the Blind
Telephone: (800) 424-8666
Web site: www.acb.org/affiliates/index.html

National Federation of the Blind of Pennsylvania
42 S. 15th Street, Suite 222
Philadelphia, PA 19102-2206
Telephone: (215) 988-0888
Web site: www.nfbp.org/states/pa.htm

Pennsylvania Association for the Blind
90 East Shady Lane
Enola, PA 17025
Telephone: (717) 234-3261
Web site: www.pablind.org/

Pennsylvania Council of the Blind
931 N. Front Street
Harrisburg, PA 17102
Telephone: (717) 920-9999 or (800) 736-1410
Web site: www.pcb1.0rg

Pennsylvania Division of Vocational Rehabilitation
444 N. Third Street, 5th Floor
Philadelphia, PA 19123
Telephone: (215) 560-1900 or (800) 442-6381
Web site: www.dli.state.pa.us

Pennsylvania Blindness and Visual Services
Philadelphia State Office Building, Room 206
1400 Spring Garden Street
Philadelphia, PA 19130-4064
Telephone: (215) 560-5700
Web site: www.dli.state.pa.us

Rhode Island

National Federation for the Blind of Rhode Island
PO Box 154564
Riverside, RI 02915
Telephone: (401) 433-2606
Web site: www.nfbri.org

Rhode Island Division of Rehabilitation Services
Office of Rehabilitation Services
40 Fountain Street
Providence, RI 02903
Telephone: (401) 421-7005 or (800) 752-8088
Web site: www.ors.ri.gov

Rhode Island Services for the Blind and Visually Impaired
40 Fountain Street
Providence, Rhode Island 02903
Telephone: (401) 222-2300
Web site: www.ors.ri.gov/SBVI.htm

South Carolina

American Council of the Blind of South Carolina
Telephone: (800) 424-8666
Web site: www.acb.org/southcarolina

National Federation for the Blind of South Carolina
1293 Professional Drive, Suite D
Myrtle Beach, SC 29577
Telephone: (803) 254-3777
Web site: www.nfbsc.net

South Carolina Commission for the Blind
PO Box 79
Columbia, SC 29202-0079
Telephone: (803) 898-8700 or (800) 922-2222
Web site: www.sccb.state.sc.us

South Carolina Division of Vocational Rehabilitation Services
State Office Building
1410 Boston Avenue
PO Box 15
West Columbia, SC 29171-0015
Telephone: (803) 896-6500
Web site: www.scvrd.net

South Dakota

American Council of the Blind of South Dakota
Telephone: (800) 424-8666
Web site: www.acb.org/affiliates/index.html

National Federation of the Blind of South Dakota
901 S. Chicago Street
Hot Springs, SD 57747
Telephone: (605) 745-5599
Web site: www.nfb.org/localorg.htm

South Dakota Association of the Blind
Telephone: (800) 424-8666
Web site: www.sd-sdab.org

South Dakota Division of Rehabilitation Services
East Highway 34, Hillsview Plaza
500 E. Capitol Avenue
Pierre, SD 57501-5070
Telephone: (605) 773-5990
Web site: www.state.sd.us/dhs/drs

South Dakota Services to the Blind and Visually Impaired
East Hwy 34500 E. Capitol
Pierre, SD 57501
Telephone: (605) 773-4644
Web site: www.state.sd.us/dhs/sbvi

Tennessee

American Council of the Blind of Tennessee
Telephone: (800) 424-8666
Web site: www.acb.org/affiliates/index.html

National Federation of the Blind of Tennessee
1226 Goodman Circle West
Memphis, TN 38111-6524
Telephone: (901) 452-6596
Web site: www.nfb.org/localorg.htm

Tennessee Department of Human Services
Services for the Blind and Visually Impaired
400 Deaderick Street, 11th Floor
Nashville, TN 37248-6200
Telephone: (615) 741-2919
Web site: www.state.tn.us/humanserv/vis-home.html

Texas

American Council of the Blind of Texas
Telephone: (800) 424-8666
Web site: www.acbtexas.org

American Foundation for the Blind–Southwest
260 Treadway Plaza, Exchange Park
Dallas, TX 75235
Telephone: (214) 352-7222
Web site: www.afb.org

National Federation of the Blind of Texas
6909 Rufus Drive
Austin, TX 78752
Telephone: (512) 323-5444
Web site: www.nfb-texas.org

Texas Commission for the Blind
4800 N. Lamar Boulevard
Austin, TX 78756-3175
Telephone: (512) 377-0500 or (800) 252-5204
Web site: www.dars.state.tx.us/dbs/index.shtml

Texas Division of Rehabilitation Services
4900 N. Lamar Boulevard
Austin, TX 78751
Telephone: (800) 628-5115
Web site: www.dars.state.tx.us/dbs

Utah

American Council of the Blind of Utah
Telephone: (800) 424-8666
Web site: www.acb.org/affiliates

National Federation of the Blind of Utah
132 Penman Lane
Bountiful, UT 84010-7634
Telephone: (801) 292-3000
Web site: www.nfbutah.org

Utah State Office of Rehabilitation
Division of Services for the Blind and Visually Impaired
250 North 1950 West, Suite B
Salt Lake City, UT 84116-7902
Telephone: (801) 323-4343 or toll-free (800) 284-1823
Web site: www.usor.utah.gov

Utah Division of Rehabilitation Services
250 E. 500 South
Salt Lake City, UT 84111
Telephone: (801) 538-7530
Web site: www.usor.utah.gov/dsbvi.htm

Vermont

American Council of the Blind of Vermont
Telephone: (800) 424-8666
Web site: www.acb.org/affiliates/index.html

National Federation of the Blind of Vermont
1 Mechanic Street, Apt. 214
Montpelier, VT 05602
Telephone: (802) 229-0748
Web site: www.nfbvt.org

Vermont Association for the Blind and Visually Impaired
37 Elmwood Avenue
Burlington, VT 05401
Telephone: (802) 863-1358
Web site: vbimail.champlain.edu

Vermont Division of Services for the Blind and Visually Impaired
103 S. Main Street
Osgood Building
Waterbury, VT 05671-2304
Telephone: (802) 241-2210
Web site: www.dad.state.vt.us

Vermont Division of Vocational Rehabilitation
162 N. Main Street
Barre, VT 05641
Telephone: (802) 479-4210 or (800) 287-2173
Web site: www.vocrehabvermont.org

Virginia

National Federation of the Blind of Virginia
Telephone: (800) 424-8666
Web site: www.nfbv.org

Old Dominion Council of the Blind and Visually Impaired
1131 S. Forest Drive
Arlington, VA 22204
Telephone: (not available)
Web site: www.acb.org/olddominion

Virginia Association of the Blind
Administrative Office
2625 Deerfield Crescent
Chesapeake, VA 23321
Telephone: (757) 465-7230
Web site: http://hometown.aol.com/vablind

Virginia Department for the Blind and Vision Impaired
397 Azalea Avenue
Richmond, VA 23227-3623
Telephone: (804) 371-3145
Web site: www.vdbvi.org

Virginia Division of Vocational Rehabilitation
202 N. Ninth Street, Suite 633
Richmond, VA 23219
Telephone: (804) 786-1201 or (800) 522-5019
Web site: www.vadrs.org/vocrehab.htm

Washington

American Council of the Blind of Washington
Telephone: (800) 424-8666
Web site: www.wcb.info

Community Services for the Blind and Partially Sighted
9709 Third Avenue NE #100
Seattle, WA 98115-2027
Telephone: (206) 525-5556 or (800) 458-4888
Web site: www.csbps.com

National Federation of the Blind of Washington
101 NE 83rd Street, Apt. A
Vancouver, WA 98665-7900
Telephone: (360) 576-5965
Web site: www.nfbw.org

Washington Division of Services for the Blind and Visually Impaired
1400 S. Evergreen Park Drive, Suite 100
Olympia, WA 98504-0933
Telephone: (360) 586-1224
Web site: www.dsb.wa.gov

Washington Division of Vocational Rehabilitation
Department of Social and Health Services
PO Box 45340
Olympia, WA 98504-5340
Telephone: (360) 438-8008 or (800) 637-5627
Web site: www1.dshs.wa.gov/dvr

Washington State Services for the Blind and Visually Impaired
800 Ninth Street SW, 4th Floor
Washington, DC 20024
Telephone: (202) 645-5869
Web site: www.dsb.wa.gov

West Virginia

Mountain State Council of the Blind
Telephone: (800) 424-8666
Web site: www.acb.org/affiliates

National Federation of the Blind of West Virginia
922 Florida Street
Milton, WV 25541-1349
Telephone: (304) 743-5114
Web site: www.nfb.org/localorg.htm

West Virginia Division of Rehabilitation Services
Blind and Visually Impaired Services
State Capitol Complex
PO Box 50890
Charleston, WV 25305
Telephone: (304) 766-4799
Web site: www.wvdrs.org

Wisconsin

Badger Association of the Blind
912 N. Hawley Road
Milwaukee WI 53213
Phone (414) 258-9200 or toll-free (877) 258-9200
Web site: www.badgerassoc.org

National Federation of the Blind of Wisconsin
2502 Elizabeth Street
Janesville, WI 53548-6711
Telephone: (608) 758-4800
Web site: www.nfbwis.org

Wisconsin Division of Rehabilitation Services
2917 International Lane, Suite 300
PO Box 7852
Madison, WI 53707-7852
Telephone: (608) 243-5603
Web site: www.dwd.state.wi.us/dvr

Wyoming

National Federation of the Blind of Wyoming
535 S. Jackson Street
Casper, WY 82601-3407
Telephone: (307) 235-9908
Web site: www.nfb.org/localorg.htm

Wyoming Council of the Blind
Telephone: (800) 424-8666
Web site: www.acb.org/affiliates

Wyoming Division of Rehabilitation Services
1100 Herschler Building, 1 East
Cheyenne, WY 82002
Telephone: (307) 777-7389
Web site: www.wyomingworkforce.org

Appendix B

AT ONE time or another, we all need help. With the high cost of medical care and prescriptions, it is good to know there is assistance for those who qualify. This is a compilation of agencies and organizations that welcome your call.

First inquire about assistance from local and state agencies:

Local—Contact a social worker at a local hospital or
community agency.
State—Find agencies listed by state in Appendix B.

If you need further help, contact these organizations:

Celebrate Sight—Coordinated by the American Academy of
Ophthalmology (AAO) offering free examinations and treatment for
glaucoma to people who do not have medical insurance.
Telephone: (800) 391-EYES (3937)
Web site: www.aao.org/public/glaucoma/gl_2001.html

Directory of Prescription Drug Patient Assistance Programs—Published by Pharmaceutical Research and Manufacturers of America, identifies company programs that provide prescription medications free of charge to physicians for their needy patients.

> Telephone: (800) PMA-INFO (762-4636)
> Address: 549 Millburn Avenue, PO Box 332, Short Hills, NJ 07078-0332
> Directory available online at www.phrma.org/patients

EyeCare America—National Eye Care Project, coordinated by the American Academy of Ophthalmology (AAO), provides free and low-cost eye exams for U.S. citizens 65 and older who have not had access to an ophthalmologist in the past three years.

> Telephone: (800) 222-EYES (3937)
> Web site: www.aao.org/public/pi/service/necp.htm

Knights Templar Eye Foundation—Provides assistance for eye surgery for people who are unable to pay or receive adequate assistance from current government agencies or similar sources.

> Telephone: (773) 205-3838
> Address: 5097 N. Elston Avenue, Suite 100, Chicago, IL 60630-2460
> Web site: www.knightstemplar.org/ktef

Lions Clubs International—Provides financial assistance for eye care through local clubs. There are Lions Clubs in most localities, and services vary from club to club. Check your telephone book for the telephone number and address of your local organization.

> Telephone of National Office: (630) 571-5466

The Medicine Program—Assists people to enroll in one or more of the many patient assistance programs that provide prescription medicine free of charge to those in need. Patients must meet the sponsor's criteria. The program is conducted in cooperation with the patient's doctor.

> Telephone: (573) 996-7300
> Address: PO Box 4182, Poplar Bluff, MO 63902-4182
> Web site: www.themedicineprogram.com

Mission Cataract USA—Coordinated nationally by the Volunteer Eye Surgeons' Association, providing free cataract surgery to people of all ages who have no other means to pay. Free eye examinations and surgeries are scheduled annually on one day, usually in May.

> Telephone: (804) 282-3931 (Virginia Eye Institute) or (800) 348-2393

New Eyes for the Needy—Provides vouchers for the purchase of new prescription eyeglasses.

> Telephone: (973) 376-4903
> Address: 549 Millburn Avenue, PO Box 332, Short Hills, NJ 07078-0332
> Web site: www.neweyesfortheneedy.org

Sight for Students—A Vision Service Plan (VSP) program in partnership with the Entertainment Industry Foundation, providing eye exams and glasses to children 18 years and younger whose families cannot afford vision care.

> Telephone: (888) 290-4964
> Web site: www.sightforstudents.org

Vision USA—Coordinated by the American Optometric Association (AOA), provides free eye care to uninsured, low-income workers and their families. Screening for the program takes place only during January of each year, with exams provided later in the year.

> Telephone: (800) 766-4466
> Address: 243 N. Lindbergh Boulevard, St. Louis, MO 63141
> Web site: www.aoa.org/visionusa/index.asp

Appendix C

Low Vision Devices

YOU HAVE read about several types of software and devices that can help you to maximize your sight and your independence. Here is contact information for some of the leading manufacturers and dealers in both optical and nonoptical products.

AbilityHub
Assistive technology for computers and disability.
c/o The Gilman Group, LLC
PO Box 6356
Rutland, VT 05702-6356
Telephone: (802) 775 1993
Web site: www.abilityhub.com

Ai Squared
For information on ZoomText® screen reader software and Big Shot Magnifier®.
PO Box 669
Manchester Center, VT 05255
Telephone: (802) 362-3612
Web site: www.aisquared.com

Allied Technologies, Inc.
Jordy® and Max® electronic magnifiers, used CCTVs, reading systems, ZoomText®.
Catalog upon request.
11440 Lakeland Drive, Suite 101
Maple Grove, MN 55369
Telephone: (800) 267-5350
Web site: www.alliedtec.com

ALVA Access Group
Windows and Macintosh access software. For information on "outSPOKEN®," text-to-speech software for Power Macintosh.
5801 Christie Avenue, Suite 475
Emeryville, CA 94608
Telephone: (510) 923-6280
Web site: www.aagi.com

ASF Lightware Solutions
ASF Magnifiers, Beam-n-Read® lights, keyboard vision aids, cell phone vision aids, playing cards, sleep switches for cassette players. Easy-to-read Web site in bold display.
Box 625
Merrick, NY 11566
Telephone: (516) 868-3918 or toll-free (800) 771-3600
Web site: www.readinglight.com

Assistive Technology, Inc.
LINK talking keyboards, computer aids, talking appliances.
7 Wells Avenue
Newton, MA 02459
Telephone: (617) 641-9000 or (800) 793-9337
Web site: www.assistivetech.com

BART Group
Adaptive hardware and software for blind and visually impaired persons. Provides onsite adaptive technology training and support along with a wide variety of products.
1489 Chain Bridge Road, Suite 104
McLean, VA 22101
Telephone: (703) 442-5023
Web site: www.bartsite.com

Bossert Specialties, Inc.
Magnification Center. Braille, CCTVs, computer and daily living aids, glasses, magnifiers, talking appliances.
3620 E. Thomas Road, Suite D-124
Phoenix, AZ 85018
Telephone: (602) 956-6637 or (800) 776-5885
Web site: www.wemagnify.com

Clarity Solutions
Products for the visually impaired. Video magnifiers.
537 College Avenue
Santa Rosa, CA 95404
Telephone: (800) 575-1456
Web site: www.clarityusa.com

Dragon Naturally Speaking
Offers a full line of multilingual speech-recognition products.
Nuance
1 Wayside Road
Burlington, MA 01803
Telephone: (781) 565-5000
Web site: www.nuance.com

Enhanced Vision
Manufacturer of Merlin®, Max®, Flipper®, Acrobat®, and Jordy® magnification systems.
Enhanced Vision Systems
17911 Sampson Lane
Huntington Beach, CA 92647
Telephone: (888) 811-3161
Web site: www.enhancedvision.com

Eschenbach Optik of America, Inc.
Vision aids include magnifiers, telescopes, sun filters, binoculars, and electronic reading devices (CCTVs).
904 Ethan Allen Highway
Ridgefield, CT 06877
Telephone: (800) 396-3886
Web site: www.eschenbach.com

Freedom Scientific

Screen reading, magnification, scanning, learning systems software. Braille note takers, embossers, and displays. Home to Arkenstone, Blazie, and Henter-Joyce.
Freedom Scientific
11800 31st Court North
St. Petersburg, FL 33716-1805
Telephone: (800) 444-4443 (U.S. and Canada)
Web site: www.freedomscientific.com

Freedom Box

An Internet accessibility product that allows disabled users to access and navigate e-mail and the Internet using voice commands.
Serotek Corporation
Telephone: (877) 661-3785
Web site: www.freedombox.info

G. W. Micro, Inc.

For information on Window Eyes®, a multifunctional speech reader program for both Windows and Macintosh. Quarterly newsletter "Focus of Vision" by subscription.
725 Airport North Office Park
Fort Wayne, IN 46825
Telephone: (219) 489-3671
Web site: www.gwmicro.com

Innoventions, Inc.

Portable electronic magnifiers Magnicam® and Primer®.
MagniCam Innoventions, Inc.
9593 Corsair Drive
Conifer, CO 80433-9317
Telephone: (303) 797-6554 or (800) 854-6554
Web site: www.magnicam.com

JBliss Low Vision Systems

Reading and magnifying systems. Imaging (scanning) software. Web browser, e-mail and word processing for low vision users. Vendor for VIP, PnC, and Web LV.
PO Box 7382
Menlo Park, CA 94026
Telephone: (888) 452-5477
Web site: www.jbliss.com

J L Ryan

Various styles of sunglasses, including BluBlocker®. Online ordering or by postal mail.
J L Ryan
216 Fry Street #5
Denton, TX 76201
Telephone: (800) 351-1265
Web site: www.jlryan.com

LazLight
High performance true-color task lamp. UV and blue light safe.
9901 NW 79th Avenue
Hialeah Gardens, FL 33016
Telephone: (305) 822-8100 or (888) 261-3738
Web site: www.lazlight.com

Low Vision Solutions
CCTVs, Quicklook®, and The View® electronic magnifiers, handheld magnifiers,
sunglasses, large-print products.
10397-A N Cherry
Kansas City, MO 64155
Telephone: (816) 734-2330 (local) or (866) 278-1850
Web site: www.lowvisionmagnification.com

LS & S Products, Inc.
Products for the visually impaired and hard of hearing. Talking and low vision prod-
ucts, computer aids, magnifiers, CCTVs, assistive technology, daily living products, and
Braille items.
PO Box 673
Northbrook, IL 60065
Telephone: (800) 468-4789
Web site: www.lssproducts.com

Maxi-Aids
Full-line catalog of blind, low vision, and products for the visually impaired, including
speech recognition, enhanced lighting, magnifiers, and talking appliances.42
Executive Boulevard
Farmingdale, NY 11735
Telephone: (516) 752-0521
Web site: www.maxiaids.com

National Association for the Visually Handicapped (NAVH)
Magnifiers, writing aids, personal items, and many more daily living aids.
22 W. 21st Street, 6th Floor
New York, NY 10010-6904
Telephone: (212) 889-3141
Web site: www.navh.org

NoIR Medical Technologies
A wide variety of UV and infrared protective sunglasses especially designed for
people with MD.
PO Box 159
South Lyon, MI 48178
Telephone: (800) 521-9746 or (734) 769-5565
Web site: www.noir-medical.com

Ocutech, Inc.
Bioptic glasses.
109 Conner Drive, Suite 2105
Chapel Hill, NC 27514-7039
Telephone: (919) 967-6460 or (800) 326-6460
Web site: www.ocutech.com

Optically Yours, Inc.
Talking watches, Corning glare control lenses, CCTVs, lighted magnifiers, electronic magnifiers, TV screen enlargers.
11797 SE U.S. Highway 441
Belleview, FL 34420-76501
Telephone: (352) 307-6797
Web site: www.opticallyyours.com

Pulse Data HumanWare, Inc.
Assistive technology in reading/writing for visual impaired. Braille, speech recognition, magnifiers.
175 Mason Circle
Concord, CA 94520
Telephone: (800) 722-3393
Web site: www.pulsedata.com

SensAbility, Inc.
Technology for reading, including CCTVs, reading machines, adaptive software, and Braille embossers.
299-B Peterson Road
Libertyville, IL 60048
Telephone: (847) 367-9009 or (888) 669-7323
Web site: not available

Sight Connection
Daily living aids for living with vision loss. Also enhanced lighting, CCTVs, and magnifiers.
Northgate Plaza
9709 Third Avenue NE, Suite 100
Seattle, CA 98115-2027
Telephone: (800) 458-4888
Web site: www.sightconnection.com

Talking Rx
Talking Rx is a simple, easy-to-use device that tells you exactly how many pills to take, when, and what for. Your doctor or pharmacist records the prescription information right into the Talking Rx.
Millennium Compliance Corp.
323 Thistle Lane
PO Box 649
Southington, CT 06489
Telephone: (888) 798-2557
Fax: (860) 426-0542
Web site: www.talkingrx.com

Telesensory Corporation
CCTVs, scanners, and video magnifiers
520 Almanor Avenue
Sunnyvale, CA 94086
Telephone: (800) 804-8004
Web site: www.telesensory.com

TextAloud®
Converts any text into voice and even to MP3.
NextUp Technologies
2539 Lewisville-Clemmons Road
Clemmons, NC 27012
Web site: www.textaloud.com

The VideoEye®
Power magnification system. This video magnification device consists of a viewing head mounted on a variable swing-arm connected to a large monitor.
VideoEye Corp.
Dept. TA
683 N. Five Mile Road
Boise, ID 83713
Telephone: (800) 416-0758
Web site: www.videoeyecorp.com

YouCan TooCan
Magnifying lamps, magnifiers, readers, clocks, telephones, talking watches, large-print products, cooking aids.
2223 S. Monaco Parkway
Denver, CO 80222
Telephone: (303) 759-9525 or toll-free (888) 663-9396
Web site: www.youcantoocan.com

Appendix D

LARGE-PRINT READING MATERIALS

MANY BOOKS and magazines are published in oversized type for people who still have usable vision. Here are leading companies in the United States that offer general reading materials in large print:

AARP
601 E Street NW
Washington, DC 20049
Telephone: (800) 424-3410
Web site: www.aarp.org

American Printing House for the Blind
1839 Frankfort Avenue
PO Box 6085
Louisville, KY 40206-0085
Telephone: (502) 895-2405 or (800) 223-1839
Web site: www.aph.org

Bibles for the Blind and Visually Handicapped International
3228 E. Rosehill Avenue
Terre Haute, IN 47805-1297
Telephone: (812) 466-4899
Web site: www.biblesfortheblind.org

Book Mountain
8851 Comanche Road
Niwot, CO 80503
Telephone: (303) 652-3950
Web site: www.bookmtn.com

Doubleday Large-Print Home Library
Membership Services Center
6550 E. 30th Street
PO Box 6325
Indianapolis, IN 46206
Telephone: (317) 541-8920
Web site: www.doubledaylargeprint.com

HarperCollins Publishers
10 E. 53rd Street
New York, NY 10022
Telephone: (212) 207-7000
Web site: www.harpercollins.com

Kensington Publishing Corp.
Dept. CO, 850 Third Avenue
New York, NY 10022
Telephone: (888) 345-2665
Web site: www.kensingtonbooks.com

The Large Print Book Company
PO Box 970
Sanbornville, NH 03872-0970
Telephone: (603) 569-4125 or (866) 569-4125
Web site: www.largeprintbookco.com

Large Print Bookshop
PO Box 5375
Englewood, CO 80155
Telephone: (303) 721-7511 or (800) 305-2743
Web site: http://members.aol.com/largeprint
(Located in the Denver Book Mall
32 N. Broadway
Denver, CO 80203)

Large Print Literary Reader
Dept. W
955 Massachusetts Avenue #105
Cambridge, MA 02139
Telephone: (617) 354-5446
Web site: www.magazinecity.net

Library of Congress
National Library Service for the Blind and Physically Handicapped
1291 Taylor Street NW
Washington, DC 20542
Telephone: (800) 424-8567 or (202) 707-5100; TDD (202) 707-0744
Web site: www.loc.gov

Library Reproduction Service
14214 S. Figueroa Street
Los Angeles, CA 90061
Telephone: (310) 354-2610 or (800) 255-5002
Web site: www.lrs-largeprint.com

New England Book Service
1037 Prindle Road
Charlotte, VT 05445
Telephone: (800) 356-5772
Web site: www.nebooks.com

The New York Times Large-Type Weekly
The New York Times
Mail Subscriptions
PO Box 9564
Uniondale, NY 11555-9564
Telephone: (800) 631-2580
Web site: www.nytimes.com

Peakirk Books
Railway Cottage 15 St. Pegas Road, Peakirk
Peterborough, CAM PE6 7NF
United Kingdom
Telephone: 011 44 1733 253182
Web site: www.abebooks.com

Random House
1540 Broadway
New York, NY 10036
Telephone: (212) 782-9000
Web site: www.randomhouse.com

Reader's Digest/Large Type Edition
PO Box 241
Mount Morris, IL 61054
Telephone: (800) 877-5293 or (815) 734-6963
Web site: www.magazinecity.net

Senior Store
629 McKinley, Suite 100
Louisville, CO 80027
Telephone: (800) 214-6849 (U.S.) or (303) 926-9301 (Non-U.S.)
Web site: www.seniorstore.com

Simon and Schuster
1230 Avenue of the Americas
New York, NY 10020
Telephone: (212} 698-7541
Web site: www.simonsays.com

Specialty Publishing and Printing
PO Box 414
Quitman, MS 39355
Telephone: (888) 697-3768
Web site: www.specialtypublishing.com

Thomas T. Beeler Publisher
710 Main Street, PO Box 310
Rollinsford, NH 03869-0310
Telephone: (800) 818-7574 or (603) 749-0392
Web site: www.beelerpub.com

Time Magazine in Large Print
PO Box 64436
Tampa, FL 33664-4436
Telephone: (914) 723-5991
Web site: www.time.com

Transaction Publishers
390 Campus Drive
Somerset, NJ 07830
Telephone: (888) 999-6778
Web site: www.transactionpub.com

The World At Large, Inc.
Biweekly newspaper with reprints of articles from *U.S. News and World Report*,
Time, the *Monitor*, and others.
1689 46th Street
Brooklyn, NY 11204
Telephone: (800) 285-2743 or (718) 972-4000
Web site: Not available

If you can't find a book you want in large print, here are companies that can specially produce it for you.

Huge Print Press
12655 N. Central Expressway, Suite 416
Dallas, TX 75243
Telephone: (866) 484-3774
Web site: www.hugeprint.com

Info Con Inc.
4550 N. Pershing Avenue, Suite 7
Stockton, CA 95207
Telephone: (209) 478-7075 or (800) 544-4551
Web site: www.infocon.com

Appendix E

DISTRIBUTORS OF AUDIOBOOKS

LISTING IN this directory is not to be considered an endorsement of the companies or their products. Neither the author nor the publisher is responsible for quality or services provided. The information is as comprehensive and accurate as possible, with the understanding that changes will occur and that not all companies could be included.

Amazon.com
Large assortment of audiobooks. Online ordering.
Web site: www.amazon.com

American Foundation for the Blind Talking Books
Information Center
11 Penn Plaza, Suite 300
New York, NY 10001
Telephone: (212) 502-7600 or (800) 232-5463
Web site: www.afb.org

American Printing House for the Blind

Free subscriptions to *Newsweek, Reader's Digest,* and other magazines. Catalog (also on cassette) listing all educational resources. Two free semiannual newsletters.
1839 Frankfort Avenue
PO Box 6085
Louisville, KY 40206-0085
Telephone: (800) 223-1839 or (502) 895-2405
Web site: www.aph.org

Assistive Media for Visually Impaired

Produces spoken-word interpretations of literary works to serve people with disabilities. These recordings are to be made easily accessible and always free of charge via the Internet.
400 Maynard Street, Suite 404
Ann Arbor, MI 48104-2434
Telephone: (734) 332-0369
Web site: www.assistivemedia.org

Associated Services for the Blind

Produces Braille, tape, and large-print materials for low vision people.
919 Walnut Street
Philadelphia, PA 19107
Telephone: (215) 627-0600 or (800) 876-5456
Web site: www.asb.org

Audible.Com

Hear your favorite public radio shows, download audiobooks, listen to your favorite newspapers, get a daily horoscope, laugh at some jokes, hear lectures, and more. Features the actor Robin Williams.
Telephone: (888) 283-5051
Web site: www.audible.com

Audiotome

A warehouse of used audiobooks.
1539 Florida Avenue
Severn, MD 21144
Telephone: (410) 551-4874
Web site: www.audiotome.com

Bible Alliance, Inc.

Scriptures in 40 languages on cassette tapes free to people with low vision.
PO Box 621
Bradenton, FL 34206
Telephone: (941) 748-3031
Web site: www.careministries.org/ba.html

Christian Record Services, Inc.
Free Christian publications and programs.
4444 S. 52nd Street
PO Box 6097
Lincoln, NE 68506
Telephone: (402) 488-0981 or TDD (402) 488-1902
Web site: www.christianrecord.org

CIL Publications and Audio Books
Created by a group of prominent rehabilitation experts, these audiobooks have
been updated to incorporate the state of the art. "We Help People Who Don't See
Well, Live Like Those Who Do."
VISIONS Services for the Blind and Visually Impaired
120 Wall Street, 16th floor
New York, NY 10005
Telephone: (888) CIL-8333
Web site: www.visionsvcb.org

Jewish Guild for the Blind
Radio reading service and books on standard cassettes.
15 W. 65th Street
New York, NY 10023
Telephone: (212) 769-6200
Web site: www.jgb.org

Jimmy B's Audio Books
A "lifetime" family membership that entitles you to rent, trade in, and purchase at a
discount.
1632 S. Pacific Coast Highway
Redondo Beach, CA 90277-5604
Telephone: (310) 792-1718
Web site: www.audiobooks.com/jimmyb/jimmyb.html

Library of Congress
Free talking book service through libraries across the country.
National Library Service for Blind and Physically Handicapped
1291 Taylor Street NW
Washington, DC 20542
Telephone: (800) 424-8567 or (202) 707-5100; TDD (202) 707-0744
Web site: www.loc.gov

Reading and Radio Resource
Free books on 2-track cassette tape or on MP-3 CD. Also operates the North Texas Radio for the Blind and records newsletters, minutes, and resource lists for various organizations.
Reading and Radio Resource
2007 Randall Street
Dallas, TX 75201
Telephone: (214) 871-7668
Web site: www.readingresource.org

Recorded Books.com
More than 2,000 audiobook titles, all unabridged, available for purchase or rent through this online site, or through our catalog. Programs for individuals, schools, and libraries.
270 Skipjack Road
Prince Frederick, MD 20678
Telephone: (800) 638-1304
Web site: www.recordedbooks.com

Regional and Sub Regional Libraries for the Blind and Physically Handicapped
Addresses of State Libraries in the U.S.A.
National Library Service for the Blind and Physically Handicapped
1291 Taylor St, NW
Washington, DC 20011
Telephone: (202) 707-5100 or toll-free (888) NLS-READ
Web site: www.loc.gov/nls/contact.html

Sound Solutions
Sound Solutions is a first-of-its kind audiocassette series that presents practical information, resources, and encouragement for seniors like you or your loved one who are experiencing sight loss.
Braille Institute
741 N. Vermont Avenue
Los Angeles, CA 90029
Telephone: (323) 663-1111 or (800) BRAILLE (272-4553)
Web site: www.biasoundsolutions.org

Tape Ministries NW
A lending library of recorded wholesome, inspirational books and spiritually uplifting devotional material serving persons who are blind, visually impaired, and physically or developmentally disabled.
Tape Ministries NW
122 SW 150th Street
Burien, WA 98166-1956
Telephone: (206) 243-7377
Web site: www.tapeministries.org

Thorndike Press
World's leading publisher of large-print books, printing more than 1,500 new titles annually.
295 Kennedy Memorial Drive
Waterville, ME 04901
Telephone: (800) 223-1244
Web site: www.gale.com

Xavier Society for the Blind
Religious and inspirational materials.
154 E. 23rd Street
New York, NY 10010
Telephone: (212) 473-7800 or (800) 637-9193
Web site: (not available)

Appendix F

DRUGS AND SUPPLEMENTS WITH ADVERSE EFFECTS ON OPHTHALMIC CONDITIONS

THIS INFORMATION was summarized from the National Registry of Drug-Induced Ocular Side Effects. For the complete report, see www.eyedrugregistry.com, or contact Casey Eye Institute, 3375 SW Terwilliger Boulevard, Portland, OR 97201-4197.

Drugs Listed

Pamidronate disodium (Aredia)
Topiramate (Topamax)
10% Phenylephrine pledgets (Neo-Synephrine)
Sildenafil (Viagra)Isotretinoin (Accutane)
Amiodarone (Cordarone)
Hydroxychloroquine/Chloroquine (Plaquenil)
Carbonic Anhydrase Inhibitors:
    Acetazolamide (Diamox)
    Dichlorphenamide (Daranide)
    Methazolamide (Glauctabs and Neptazane)
Topical Ocular Dorzolamide (Trusopt)

Topical Ocular Prostaglandin Analogs:
- Travoprost (Travatan)
- Latanoprost (Xalatan)
- Bimatoprost (Lumigan)
- Unoprostone isopropyl (Rescula)

Pamidronate disodium (Aredia)

Primary Use: The class of drugs called bisphosphonates inhibits bone resorption in the management of hypercalcemia of malignancy, osteolytic bone metastases of both breast cancer and multiple myeloma, and Paget's disease of the bone. These drugs are also used in the treatment of osteoporosis. Other bisphosphonates are alendronic acid (Fosamax), ibandronate, zolendronate (Zometa), risedronate sodium (Actonel), and clodronate (Bonefos).

Certain side effects:
- Blurred vision
- Ocular irritation
- Nonspecific conjunctivitis
- Pain
- Epiphoria

Photophobia
- Anterior Uveitis (rare—posterior)
- Anterior Scleritis (rare—posterior)
- EpiscleritisPeriocular, lid and/or orbital edema

Possible side effects:
- Retrobulbar neuritis
- Yellow vision
- Diplopia
- Cranial nerve palsy
- Ptosis
- Visual hallucinations

Topiramate (Topamax)

Primary Use: Topiramate is a novel agent used in various types of epilepsy, migraine headaches, depression, neuropathic pain, and bipolar disorders. It is used off label as a "magic" weight reduction medication.

Certain side effects:
  Acute glaucoma (angle closure)
  Anterior shallowing
  Decreased vision
  Ocular pain
  Headaches
  Ocular hyperemia
  Mydriasis—variable or absent
  Uveitis
  Visual field defects
  Myopia (up to 6–8 diopters)
  Suprachoroidal effusions

Probable/Likely side effects:
  Blepharospasm
  Oculogyric crisis

Possible side effects:
  Retinal bleeds
  Scleritis
  Teratogenic—ocular malformations

10% Phenylephrine pledgets (Neo-Synephrine)

Primary Use: Hemostasis during LASIK procedures, potentiate pupillary dilation, lyse posterior synechiae.

Certain side effects:
  Hypertension

Probable/Likely side effects:
  Myocardial infarction
  Subarachnoid **hemorrhage**

Sildenafil (Viagra)

Primary Use: Management of erectile dysfunction.

Certain side effects:
Changes in color perception
Objects have colored tinges—usually blue or blue/green, may be pink or yellow
Diminished color vision (Farnsworth-Munsell 100 Hue Test)
Dark colors appear darker
Blurred vision
Central haze
Transitory decreased vision
Changes in light perception
Increased perception of brightness
Flashing lights—especially when blinking
ERG changes
Conjunctival hyperemia
Photophobia

Possible side effects (could be secondary, not directly drug-related):
Mydriasis
Anterior ischemic optic neuropathy
Retinal vascular accidents

Isotretinoin (Accutane)

Primary Use: Treatment of cystic acne, psoriasis, and various skin disorders.

Certain side effects:
Abnormal meibomian gland secretion
Meibomian gland **atrophy**
Blepharoconjunctivitis
Myopia
Corneal opacities
Ocular discomfort
Decreased dark adaptation
Ocular sicca
Decreased tolerance for contact lenses

Photophobia
Decreased vision
Increased tear osmolarity
Teratogenic ocular abnormalities
Keratitis
Teratogenic ocular abnormalities

Probable/Likely side effects:
Decreased color vision (reversible)
Permanent loss of dark adaptation
Pseudotumor cerebri

Possible side effects:
Corneal ulcers
Optic neuritis
Diplopia
Permanent sicca-like syndrome
Eyelid edema
Subconjunctival hemorrhage
Idiopathic intracranial hypertension with optic disk edema

Unlikely side effects:
Activation of herpes simplex virus
Keratoconus
Corneal vascularization
Limbal infiltrates
Exophthalmos
Pupil abnormalities
Glaucoma
Vitreous disturbance

Conditional/Unclassifiable side effects:
Cataracts
Peripheral field loss
Cortical blindness
Retinal findings
Decreased accommodation
Scleritis
Iritis

Amiodarone (Cordarone)

Primary Use: Treatment of various cardiac arrhythmias.

Certain side effects:
Photosensitivity
Corneal microdeposits
Visual sensations:
Hazy vision
Colored halos around lights
Bright lights
Glare
Aggravates sicca (dry eyes)
Periocular skin pigmentation
Blepharoconjunctivitis
Thyroid eye disease

Probable side effects:
Corneal ulceration
Interior subcapsular lens opacities
Nonarteritic ischemic optic neuropathy
Loss of eyelashes or eyebrows
Pseudotumor cerebri

Possible side effects:
Autoimmune reaction (dry mouth, dry eyes, peripheral neuropathy, and pneumonitis)
Amiodarone-induced optic neuropathy
Nonarteritic anterior ischemic optic neuropathy

Hydroxychloroquine/Chloroquine (Plaquenil)*

Primary Use: Treatment of rheumatoid arthritis and lupus erythematosis, dermatologic conditions, and various inflammatory disorders.

---

* Chloroquine is no longer available except for malaria treatment, primarily military.

Side effects:
    Scotomas
    Retinal changes
    Color vision loss
    Decreased vision

Carbonic Anhydrase Inhibitors (CAI)

Acetazolamide (Diamox), dichlorphenamide (Daranide), methazolamide (Glauctabs and Neptazane)

Primary Use: Oral sales of CAI. Short-term use in cataract surgery, prevention of air hunger in mountain climbers, use in selected cases of macular edema, and as an ocular pressure–lowering drug.

Side effects:
    CAI may significantly increase respiratory distress in chronic lung disease patients.
    Causes osteomalacia in patients on anticonvulsive medication.
    Patients on high doses of aspirin plus CAI can experience aspirin-induced CNS toxicity.
    Can cause metabolic acidosis and coma, especially in patients with renal insufficiency or diabetics with nephropathy.
    Patients with cirrhosis can get ammonia poisoning.
    Stevens-Johnson syndrome—Japanese appear to be more susceptible.
    Concomitant use of CAI may increase five-fold trough blood levels of cyclosporine with pronounced nephro- and neurotoxicity.

Topical Ocular Dorzolamide (Trusopt)

Primary Use: Treatment of glaucoma.

Side Effects:
    Bitter, metallic-like taste.
    Increased salivation.
    Tongue and perioral numbness and edema.

Various gastrointestinal complaints, such as nausea, abdominal cramping, heartburn and upset stomach (occurring in up to 10% of patients). Rare: headaches, fatigue, insomnia, depression.

Topical Ocular Prostaglandin Analogs

Travoprost (Travatan), latanoprost (Xalatan), bimatoprost (Lumigan), unoprostone isopropyl (Rescula)

Primary Use: Pressure-lowering agents, singularly or as an additive.

Side effects:

Increased iris pigmentation, especially in irides brown at the pupillary border and hazel or blue peripherally, with greatest color change in relatively hypopigmented irises.

Increased pigmentation due to increased melanin within each melanocyte, rather than hyperplasia.

Increased pigmentation of eyelashes and periorbital skin. Some skin hypopigmentation has been reported, but cannot as yet prove this is drug-related.

Eyelash curling.

Increased hair growth in eyelashes and adjacent adnexal hair.

Low-grade iritis or uveitis, especially in patients with prior history of uveitis or incisional ocular surgery.

In glaucoma patients with a history of uveitis, latanoprost may cause an increase in intraocular pressure and a recurrence of intraocular inflammation.

Macular edema—including cystoid macular edema. Associated usually with uveitis.

Most common in aphakic eyes, especially with torn posterior capsules. Also more common in patients with known risks for macular edema.

In long-term use, may cause pigmentary glaucoma in younger patients.

May aggravate herpes simplex keratits and periocular herpes simplex dermatitis.

May cause migraine headaches.

May cause iris **cysts**.

May impair precorneal tear film stability.

Overview comparison of ocular side effects of these 4 prostaglandin analogs:

Probably no known systemic side effects to date.

Bimatoprost and travoprost have the highest frequency and severity of hyperemia and eyelash growth, compared to latanoprost and timinol.

Frequency of color darkening between bimatoprost, travoprost and latanoprost is the same.

Unoprostone can produce punctate keratopathy.

More headaches reported with latanoprost than with bimatoprost.

Systemic side effects:

Flulike symptoms (abdominal cramps, malaise and URI).

Four reports of aggravated asthma.

Question of increased migraine headaches.

Rare reports of angina, arterial hypertension, or tachycardia.

Appears to be a very safe drug systemically, but no long-term studies have been accomplished at this time.

Supplements

The following supplements have been found to have a wide range of adverse ocular side effects ranging from dry eye to retinal hemorrhages and transient visual loss:

ginkgo biloba
echinacea purpurea
chamomile, licorice
canthaxanthine
datura (jimson weed)
niacin and vitamin A

This was reported by Frederick W. Fraunfelder, MD (Oregon Health and Science University researcher) to the World Health Organization, the U.S. Food and Drug Administration, and the National Registry of Drug-Induced Ocular Side Effects. For more information, see the October 2004 issue of the *American Journal of Ophthalmology*.

Glossary of Terms Related to Retinal Disease

ACUITY: Level of clarity, distinction, or sharpness.

ACUITY TEST: Use of an eye chart to measure accuracy of reading and perception at various distances. (*See* "Snellen visual acuity chart.")

AQUEOUS CHAMBER: The space directly behind the cornea, filled with a clear fluid for the purpose of maintaining the pressure of the eye.

AFTERIMAGE: Continued visual perception after the source of the image has been removed.

AGE-RELATED MACULAR DEGENERATION: A progressive disease of the central part of the retina (the macula) usually affecting adults age 60 and older, in which the light-sensing cells wither from aging and may lead to central vision loss.

ALTERNATIVE TREATMENT (ALSO "ALTERNATIVE MEDICINE." ALSO "COMPLEMENTARY" TREATMENT OR MEDICINE): Outside of the realm of clinically proven intervention or generally accepted protocol in the medical field.

AMBLYOPIA: Diminished vision in one or both eyes without apparent physical reason, and despite best lens correction.

AMSLER GRID: A grid chart used for checking distortion in vision and central vision defects.

ANESTHESIA: A drug-induced (anesthetic) decreased sensitivity to pain.

ANEURYSM: Localized, pathological, blood-filled dilatations of a blood vessel caused by a disease or weakening of the vessel's wall.

ANGIOGENESIS: New blood vessel growth.

ANTERIOR: The front or forward portion.

ANTIANGIOGENIC: A general term for drugs that have the capability of preventing new vessel growth (neovascularization) in the retina.

ANTIOXIDANTS: Substances produced by the body that counteract the effects of free radicals. Present in dark green, leafy vegetables such as spinach and kale, and may also be acquired through supplements such as vitamins C, E, and carotenoids, including beta-carotene.

AREDS: Age-Related Eye Disease Study, which recommended high dosages of certain antioxidant vitamins and zinc for early stage AMD patients.

ARGON LASER: Laser light produced from argon gas. Nine separate wavelengths in the blue-green visible light spectrum are produced, but the main wavelengths are 488.0 nm blue and 514.5 nm pea-green light.

ASYMPTOMATIC: No symptoms present.

ATROPHIC MACULAR DEGENERATION: "Dry" macular degeneration.

ATROPHY: A wasting of the tissue due to loss of nutrition or neural stimulus.

AUTOMATED PERIMETER: A computer-driven device used to plot defects in the visual field.

AUTOSOMAL DOMINANT: A trait or disease that is produced when only one copy of a gene is present.

AUTOSOMAL RECESSIVE: A trait or disease that is produced only when two copies of a gene are present.

BEST CORRECTED VISUAL ACUITY: A measure of best focus while wearing corrective lenses.

BETA-BLOCKER: A drug (e.g., thalidomide) that inhibits the growth of blood vessels. Currently being studied as a cancer cure, with possible benefits in the field of macular degeneration.

BETA-CAROTENE: A yellow photopigment chemical synthesized by plants and present in vitamin A.

BILATERAL: Referring to both eyes.

BINOCULAR VISION: Blending of the separate images seen by the two eyes. Normal binocular vision produces a stereoscopic image and parallax-induced depth perception.

BLIND: A condition of the retina resulting in no sensory response to light.

BLIND SPOT: A natural area of no vision in the outer periphery where the optic nerve enters the eye. Also, an area of no vision as a result of degenerated photoreceptor cells. (*See* "scotoma.")

BLUE LIGHT: Potentially hazardous light rays that are near ultraviolet (400–500 nm) and which cause production of free radicals in the retinal cells.

BRACHYTHERAPY: Radiation treatment delivered by a small plaque sewn to the sclera.

BRAILLE: A system of raised dots on a page representing letters and words, invented by Louis Braille.

BRIGHTNESS ACUITY TESTER (BAT): A device which analyzes a patient's ability to see under glare conditions, such as bright daylight.

BRUCH'S MEMBRANE (OR LAYER): The innermost membrane of the choroid layer within the retina. The lamina vitrea.

CAROTENOIDS: Photochemical and photosensitive agents in plants and animals, composed of fat-soluble, highly unsaturated pigmented organic chemicals.

CARRIER: An individual with one mutated gene paired with one normal gene. A carrier of a gene for a recessive disease does not have the disease.

CATARACT: A clouding of the crystalline lens of the eye or its surrounding transparent membrane, obstructing the passage of light and causing a reduction in vision.

CELL: The smallest unit of living matter. The human body is made up of about ten trillion cells.

CENTRAL RETINAL ARTERY: The vessel that delivers blood into the eye and supplies nutrients to the retina.

CENTRAL RETINAL VEIN: The vessel that carries blood away from the retina.

CERTIFIED LOW VISION THERAPIST (CLVT): A person who is trained to work in conjunction with optometrists and ophthalmologists in the implementation of a low vision patient's evaluation and training.

CHARLES BONNET SYNDROME (CBS): A nonpsychotic condition seen in low vision people, wherein often pleasant and harmless hallucinations occur.

CHOROID: The layer of the eye behind the retina containing blood vessels that nourish the inner cell layers.

CHROMOSOME: A microscopic, rodlike structure in the cell's nucleus that carries genetic material.

CLASSIC: A type of wet macular degeneration wherein the leaking blood vessels are identifiable under magnification.

CLINICAL DEPRESSION: A physical/mental state of depression that meets the criteria accepted by most clinicians and that lasts two weeks or longer.

CLINICAL TESTING (OR TRIAL): Direct observation of a living patient to answer specific questions about vaccines, therapies, or new methods.

COLOR VISION: The ability to perceive differences in color, including hue, saturation, and brightness.

COMPLICATION: An undesirable effect of a disease or its treatment.

COMPUTERIZED PERIMETERS TEST: An examination wherein the doctor uses a computer to present lights or other targets in various positions and map out the field loss areas.

CONE CELLS: The photoreceptor cells in the retina that are responsible for central and color vision under bright conditions (photopic focal points).

CONFRONTATIONS TEST: An examination where the doctor moves his hand or lights in from the side to see if there is any loss of peripheral vision due to stroke.

CONTRAST SENSITIVITY: The ability to differentiate between an object and its background.

CONTROL GROUP: That segment of an experimental study population that receives a sham, or fake, treatment.

CORNEA: The transparent part of the eyeball that covers the iris and pupil.

CUP/DISC RATIO: The area of the level part of the optic disc divided by the area of the deep part, or cup, of the optic disc.

CYST: A membrane sac containing fluid or semisolid matter.

DEGENERATION: Deterioration as a result of chemical change or invasion of abnormal matter.

DEPTH PERCEPTION: The ability to judge the relative distance of objects and the spatial relationship of objects at different distances.

DIAGNOSIS: The name of a disease or condition.

DILATION: The process wherein the pupil automatically enlarges to allow more light to reach the retina. Also, chemically induced enlargement of the pupil by a doctor to allow easier examination of the interior of the eye.

DISCIFORM AMD: The disciform (wet) type of macular degeneration involving neovascularization.

DISEASE: An abnormal and troubling mental or physical condition.

DNA: Deoxyribonucleic acid, the molecule that holds genetic information. It is the biochemical molecule that makes chromosomes and genes.

DOMINANT EYE: The eye that looks directly at an object, while the nondominant eye views it from the side.

DOUBLE IMAGE (OR "DIPLOPIA"): A second image (usually dimmer) caused by the eyes not aiming equally on an object. Also called "ghosting."

DOUBLE-BLIND (MORE APPROPRIATELY "DOUBLE-MASKED"): A type of experiment in which neither the subject nor the administrator knows whether the test treatment is real or fake.

DOSE-ESCALATION (ALSO "DOSE-RANGING"): An experiment wherein all subjects receive the treatment in different amounts of a drug to test for safety and efficacy.

DRUSEN: Small, yellowish, protein lipid deposits in the retina appearing in the early stages of dry (atrophic) macular degeneration. Two types: hard and soft, with the latter being more likely to signal future retinal problems.

DRY EYE SYNDROME: A condition in which the tear ducts do not supply sufficient moisture to the eyeball, resulting in sensations of pain and stinging.

DRY MACULAR DEGENERATION (ALSO "ATROPHIC" MACULAR DEGENERATION): The form of macular degeneration wherein the retinal cone cells degenerate due to age.

DYSTROPHY: Degeneration, abnormal or defective development, insufficient nutrition.

EARLY-ONSET MACULAR DEGENERATION: (*see* "juvenile macular degeneration")

ECCENTRIC VIEWING: The practice of seeing peripherally as a substitute for loss of central vision.

EDEMA: An abnormal excess accumulation of fluid in a tissue.

ENZYME: A protein involved in an important biochemical reaction in the body. A defective enzyme can be the result of a mutated gene.

EXPERIMENTAL GROUP: That segment of an experimental study population that receives the treatment being tested.

EXUDE: To discharge moisture.

EXTRAFOVEAL: Outside of the fovea, or very center of the macula.

EYE: The organ of sight. Spheroid in shape, approximately one inch in diameter.

FDA: Abbreviation for the United States Food and Drug Administration. Responsible for approving and regulating treatments, procedures, and pharmaceuticals.

FIGURE-GROUND PERCEPTION: The ability to differentiate images from the background.

FLASHER: An illusion of flashing light created when the vitreous gel, which fills the inside of the eye, rubs or pulls on the retina.

FLOATERS: Small clumps of vitreous gel or cellular debris in the vitreous fluid.

FLUORESCEIN ANGIOGRAM (FA): A procedure for viewing and photographing the inner eye involving injection of a nontoxic dye into the bloodstream.

FOVEA: The concave center of the retina. The region of highest visual acuity and cone cell density.

FREE RADICALS: Atoms with single missing electrons that cause cellular damage by taking electrons from molecules in healthy cells. This process is called oxidation.

FUNDUS PHOTO: Image of the back of the eye.

GENE REPLACEMENT THERAPY: The procedure of introducing a nondefective gene into the body to take the place of a defective one.

GLARE: Intense light into the eyes causing discomfort.

GLAUCOMA: A condition in which the pressure inside the eye increases beyond the norm, damaging the optic nerve and causing loss of peripheral vision.

HEADACHE (OCULAR): Cranial pain thought to result from eye disease or excessive use.

HEMORRHAGE: Leaking of blood from the vessels.

HYPERTENSION: High blood pressure. Possibly—but

not proven to be—linked to the wet form of macular degeneration.

HYPEROPIA (OR FARSIGHTEDNESS): A condition in which rays of light from nearby objects are focused behind the retina, causing blurred vision.

HYPOXIA: A deficiency of oxygen supply to a tissue.

IDIOPATHIC: A disease having no known cause.

ILLUMINATION (OR "ILLUMINANCE"): A light source. Scientifically, the amount of flux per unit area on a lighted surface.

INDOCYANINE GREEN ANGIOGRAPHY: Photography of the retina using a green dye that fluoresces under ultraviolet light.

INFECTION: Spreading of microorganisms throughout bodily tissue or parts.

INFORMED CONSENT: The process of learning key facts about a clinical trial before participating, including:
    why the study is being done
    what is to be accomplished
    what will be done and for how long
    what risks are involved
    what benefits can be expected
    what other treatments are available
    whether the subject may quit the trial at any time

INFUSION: Introduction of fluid into the body by gravity through an intravenous (IV) tube.

INHERITANCE PATTERN: The way in which a gene or trait is passed through generations of a family.

INJECTION: Introduction of fluid into the body by forced penetrance with a needle and syringe.

INTRAOCULAR: Inside the eyeball.

INTRAOCULAR LENS (IOL): An artificial replacement for the eye's natural lens.

INTRAVITREAL: Within the vitreous fluid of the eyeball.

IRIS: The colored diaphragm in the anterior chamber of the eyeball that contracts and expands to adjust for light intensity.

IRRADIATE: To expose to radiation for diagnostic or therapeutic purposes.

JUVENILE MACULAR DEGENERATION (ALSO "EARLY-ONSET MACULAR DEGENERATION"): Progressive diseases of the macula that are usually inherited, affecting children, teenagers and young adults.

JUXTA: Next to, as in juxtafoveal and juxtascleral.

LASER PHOTOCOAGULATION: An outpatient treatment wherein blood vessels are cauterized by the heat from a fine-point laser beam.

LEGAL BLINDNESS: A standard of visual acuity set at 20/200 with correction in the better eye (*see* "Snellen chart") or a visual field of less than 20 degrees.

LENS: The transparent, dual-convex body that focuses light rays onto the retina.

LINKED: Two or more markers that are close enough together on a chromosome to be inherited together.

LIPOFUSCIN: Fatty deposits in the retina that are thought to be toxic to retinal cells. A by-product of drusen.

LOW VISION (OR VISUALLY IMPAIRED): Significantly impaired vision that is not correctable with conventional devices.

LOW VISION DEVICES: Equipment designed to allow improved vision, usually by magnification.

LOW VISION REHABILITATION: Training for the visually impaired in adaptability and in the use of low vision devices, computer software, and motility aids.

LOW VISION SPECIALIST: An optometrist who has been specially trained in the examination, treatment, and management of patients with impaired vision.

LOW VISION THERAPIST: A person who is certified to assist eye care specialists in providing training for visually-impaired people.

MACULA (ALSO "MACULA LUTEA," OR "YELLOW MACULA"): The center of vision, containing mostly cone cells for detail, color, and daytime viewing.

MACULAR DEGENERATION: A disease of the central part of the retina (the macula) in which the cells wither, leading to loss of central vision. (*Also see* "Age-related" and "juvenile" macular degeneration.)

MACULAR TRANSLOCATION: A surgical procedure wherein the macula is rotated slightly to a healthier part of the retina.

MARKER: A gene or DNA fragment with a known location on a chromosome that is associated with a certain disease. It can be used as a point of reference when looking for disease-causing mutations.

MELANIN: The substance that gives color to the eyes and protects the macula by trapping light rays.

MEMBRANE: A thin layer of tissue that covers, surrounds, lines, or separates parts of the body.

MIGRAINE FLASHERS: (*See* "ophthalmic migraine")

MINIMALLY CLASSIC CNV: A type of wet AMD wherein the leaking blood vessels occupy half or less of the area of the entire lesion.

MUTATION: A change in a gene.

MYOPIA (ALSO "NEARSIGHTEDNESS"): A condition in which rays of light from distant objects are focused in front of the retina, causing blurred vision.

NASAL: Toward the nose.

NATURAL BLIND SPOT: An area of nonvision in the periphery of each eye caused by the absence of sight cells at the location of the optic disc.

NEOVASCULARIZATION: Growth of new, fragile blood vessels that may leak beneath the retina.

NONOPTICAL DEVICES: Equipment used for supplementing or replacing vision, such as audio tape players, scanners, etc.

NUCLEUS: The central structure within the cell, which contains genetic material.

NUTRACEUTICAL: A natural food or supplement that is beneficial to health.

O & M: Abbreviation for "orientation and mobility" training in the use of the white cane.

OCULAR COHERENCE TOMOGRAPHY (OCT): A diagnostic method that uses an optical device to generate a cross-section image of the retinal layers, allowing for measurement of tissue thickness.

OCULAR MOTILITY: Movement of the eyes in relation to one another.

OCCULT CNV: The type of subfoveal blood vessel presence in wet AMD that has a source not readily defined.

OD (*OCULUS DEXTER*): Latin abbreviation for "right eye."

OPHTHALMIC MIGRAINE (ALSO "MIGRAINE FLASHERS"): Zigzag, shimmering, or even colorful lines that sometimes move within the visual field bilaterally. Thought to be caused by a sudden spasm of blood vessels in the brain.

OPHTHALMOSCOPY: Examination of the internal structures of the eye using an illumination and magnification system.

OPHTHALMOLOGIST: A practitioner in the medical

science of surgery and care of the eye and its related structures. An MD degree is required.

OPTIC DISC: The junction of all of the retinal nerve fibers at the beginning of the optic nerve. Appears as a grayish disc shape near the fovea in fundus photos.

OPTIC NERVE: Transmits neural impulses from the retinal cell layers to the brain.

OPTICIAN: A person who designs or manufactures ophthalmic appliances or optical instruments ("ophthalmic optician") or deals in prescriptions ("dispensing optician").

OPTOMETRIST: An independent, primary health care provider who is skilled in the comanagement of eye health and vision care, to include examination, diagnosis, treatment, management of diseases and disorders, prescription of eyeglasses and contact lenses, and provision of low vision aids and vision therapy. An OD degree is required.

OS (*OCULUS SINISTER*): Latin abbreviation for "left eye."

OU (*OCULI UNITER, OR UNITAS*): Latin abbreviation meaning both eyes working simultaneously as a unit.

OXIDATION: Loss of electrons from molecules in healthy cells, caused by free radicals and leading to loss of vision.

PATHOLOGICAL: Caused by or having to do with a disease.

PEDIGREE: A multigenerational family tree using symbols to denote lineage and genetic information.

PERIPHERAL VISION: The outer part of the field of vision made possible by the rod cells.

PHARMACEUTICAL: A substance, such as a drug or medicine, used in medical treatment.

PHOTODYNAMIC THERAPY (PDT): The process of

blood vessel coagulation in the retina through activation of a light-sensitive drug injected into the system.

PHOTOPHOBIA: Sensitivity to light.

PHOTORECEPTOR: a retinal cell that converts light into nerve impulses, which are then processed by the retina and sent through nerve fibers to the brain.

PLACEBO: An inactive substance that has no effect on the body.

PLURIPOTENT: Stem cells that have the potential to develop into a number of different cell types, such as red blood cells, platelets, or lymphocytes.

POLARIZATION: A process whereby a chemical film is applied to glass to reduce horizontal glare (e.g., reflection off water or roadways).

POSTERIOR: Behind, or the back surface.

POSTERIOR VITREOUS DETACHMENT (PVD): Separation of the vitreous gel from the retina.

PREDOMINANTLY CLASSIC CNV: A type of wet AMD wherein the leaking vessels are well defined.

PREFERRED RETINAL LOCUS (PRL): The favored fixation point for viewing an image.

PROGENITOR CELL (ALSO "ADULT STEM CELL"): A type of stem cell that is more developed than a completely unspecialized embryonic stem cell.

PROSTHESIS: An artificial device that replaces a missing part of the body.

PROTEINS: Large organic molecules that are made up of all of the basic substances of the body.

PUPIL: The opening in the center of the iris through which light passes.

REDUCED PENETRANCE: A gene whose effect has been modified or reduced.

RETINA: The cell layers on the inner wall of the eyeball that convert light from the lens into nerve impulses for delivery to the brain through the optic nerve.

RETINAL CELL LAYERS: The membrane on the inner wall of the eyeball that receives the image from the lens and converts it into neural impulses.

RETINAL PIGMENT EPITHELIUM (RPE): A single layer of cells lying between the photoreceptor cells and the choroid layer. The RPE delivers nourishment to the photoreceptors.

RETINA SPECIALIST: A medical doctor who specializes in diseases such as retinal detachments, advanced diabetic retinopathy, and some forms of macular degeneration.

RETINAL TEAR: A rip in the retinal tissue caused by pulling (traction) of the vitreous gel where the two are joined.

RETINAL DETACHMENT: Separation of the retina from its connection at the back of the eyeball, usually caused by a retinal tear.

RNA (RIBONUCLEIC ACID): A molecule, similar to DNA, which carries information into the cell from DNA to synthesize proteins.

ROD CELLS: The photoreceptor cells in the retina that are responsible for peripheral and night vision (scotopic focal points).

RUYSCHIAN MEMBRANE: A network of capillaries in the choroid that supplies the outer five retinal layers. This network is most dense at the macula.

SCANNING LASER OPHTHALMOSCOPY (SLO): A device for photographing the retina, wherein a quickly scanning low-intensity laser sends images to a computer monitor.

SCLERA: The white, dense, fibrous outer coating of the eyeball.

SCLERAL BUCKLE: A surgical procedure for high myopes that inhibits further stretching of the eyeball.

SCOTOMA: A blind spot, or area of diminished sensitivity in the visual field.

SCOTOPIC VISION: Night vision.

SEX CHROMOSOME: An X or Y chromosome. The XX pair determines female, and the XY pair determines male.

SHAM: A fake treatment or drug administered to the control group in an experimental study.

SLIT LAMP: An instrument with a light source that is focused into a slit for use, in combination with a biomicroscope, in examining the frontal structures of the eye.

SMALL INTERFERENCE RNA (siRNA): A drug that blocks VEGF from forming by turning off the gene that produces it.

SNELLEN VISUAL ACUITY CHART: The standard tool for the measurement of visual acuity, displaying letters of progressively smaller size.

STATIN: A type of cholesterol-reducing drug that lowers the levels of fats (lipids) in the blood.

STEM CELLS: Undeveloped structures that are able develop into any of the nearly 220 cell types that make up the human body and that can theoretically reproduce themselves infinitely.

STEREOPSIS: The capability of depth perception in both eyes.

SUBCUTANEOUS: Beneath the skin.

SUBFOVEAL: Beneath the fovea.

SURGICAL: A medical procedure involving an incision or laser procedure.

SYMPTOMATIC: Displaying symptoms.

SYNDROME: A group of symptoms that identify a particular disease or condition.

TANGENT SCREEN TEST: An examination during which the patient identifies a spot of light moving into his peripheral field.

TEAR FILM: The clear saline fluid that cleanses and lubricates the front surface of the eye.

TEMPORAL: Toward the ear.

ULTRASONOGRAPHY (ULTRASOUND): The use of sound waves to examine the eye and surrounding area for analysis of tumors, retinal detachments, or cataracts.

ULTRAVIOLET (UV): Light wavelengths that are shorter than the violet end of the visible spectrum and longer than the roentgen radiations.

VARIABLE EXPRESSIVITY: A gene whose effect varies from one person to the next.

VEGF (VASCULAR ENDOTHELIAL GROWTH FACTOR): A protein that is responsible for blood vessel development (**ANGIOGENESIS**).

VIP: Visually impaired person.

VIRAL (VIRUS) VECTOR: An agent developed from a virus used to transport a replacement gene into the body.

VISION REHABILITATION SPECIALIST: A person who is certified to instruct the visually impaired in management of daily living activities.

VISUAL FIELD: The area that can be seen by one immobile eye.

VISUAL FIELD GRID: A variation of the Amsler grid that tests both distortion and blind areas in the vision.

VISUALLY IMPAIRED (OR LOW VISION): Significantly impaired vision that is not correctable with conventional devices.

VITRECTOMY: An operation designed to remove diseased vitreous and repair or protect the retina.

VITREOUS FLUID (ALSO VITREOUS "GEL" OR "HUMOR"): A clear jelly-like substance that fills the posterior chamber of the eyeball.

WET (EXUDATIVE OR NEOVASCULAR) MACULAR DEGENERATION: The form of macular degeneration involving neovascularization and leakage into the subretinal space.

Notes

1. These figures were derived from a presentation given to the 2002 ARVO convention by researchers from the Wilmer Eye Institute, Johns Hopkins University, and 20RC Macro International. For more information, see www.mdsupport.org/library/numbers.html.
2. Definition of "disease," in *The American Heritage Stedman's Medical Dictionary* (Houghton Mifflin, 2002).
3. For more information about color perception, see www.mdsupport.org/library/color.html.
4. This information is based upon the article by Wendy Strouse Watt, OD, "How Visual Acuity Is Measured," MD Support Library 2003: www.mdsupport.org/library.html.
5. The normal height for the letter A is 88 millimeters, and the viewing distance is 6 meters. The distance here is calculated by dividing the height of the letter A (31.75mm) by 88 and multiplying the result by 6.
6. To view photographs of AMD patients' visual perceptions based upon results from the visual field grid, see www.mdsupport.org/thrueyes.html.
7. J. M. Seddon, et al., "Progression of Age-Related Macular Degeneration: Association with Body Mass Index, Waist Circumference, and Waist-Hip Ratio," *Archives of Ophthalmology* 121, no. 6 (2003): 785–92.

8. B. E. Klein, R. Klein, L. E. Lee, et al., "Measures of Obesity and Age-Related Eye Diseases," *Ophthalmic Epidemiology* 8, no. 4 (2001): 251–62.

9. Judy McBride, "Can Foods Forestall Aging? Some with High Antioxidant Activity Appear to Aid Memory," Jean Mayer USDA Human Nutrition Research Center on Aging, *Agricultural Research* 47, no. 2 (February 1999): 15–17.

10. Floyd H. Chilton, PhD, *Inflammation Nation: The First Clinically Proven Eating Plan to End Our Nation's Secret Epidemic* (New York: Fireside, 2004), 320.

11. Ellen Troyer, MT, MA, "Of Mice, Men, and Omega 6 Arachidonic Acid (AA)," Friday Pearl, BioSyntrx, Inc. (May 6, 2005).

12. Health and Welfare Canada, "Nutrition Recommendations: The Report of the Scientific Review Committee," Department of Supply and Services Cat. No.H49-42/1990E (1990), Ottawa, ON.

13. J. M. Seddon, et al., "NIH Eye Disease Case-Control Study," *Journal of the American Medical Association* 272 (1994): 1413–20.

14. Stuart Richer, OD, PhD, et al., "The LAST study (Lutein Antioxidant Supplementation Trial)," *Optometry—The Journal of the American Optometric Association* 75, no. 4 (April 2004): 216–29.

15. Recommended by the Centers for Disease Control (CDC).

16. C. R. Gale, N. F. Hall, et al., "Lutein and Zeaxanthin Status and Risk of Age-Related Macular Degeneration," *Investigative Ophthalmology and Visual Science* 44, no. 6 (June 2003): 2461–65.

17. Author unkown, "Lutein and Zeaxanthin—a Scientific Review," Roche Vitamins (2001).

18. U.S. Department of Agriculture, Agricultural Research Service, USDA Nutrient Data Laboratory, USDA National Nutrient Database for Standard Reference (2004)

19. Ki Won Lee, et al., "Cocoa Has More Phenolic Phytochemicals and a Higher Antioxidant Capacity than Teas and Red Wine," *Journal of Agricultural and Food Chemistry* 51, no. 25 (December 2003): 7292–95.

20. Age-Related Eye Disease Study Research Group, "A Randomized, Placebo-Controlled, Clinical Trial of High-Dose Supplementation with Vitamins C and E, Beta Carotene, and Zinc for Age-Related Macular Degeneration and Vision Loss: AREDS Report No. 8," *Archives of Ophthalmology* 119, no. 10 (October 2001): 1417–36.

21. J. Feher, A. Papale, et al., "Improvement of Visual Functions and Fundus Alterations in Early Age-Related Macular Degeneration Treated with a Combination of Acetyl-L-Carnitine, N-# Fatty Acids, and Coenzyme Q10. *Ophthalmologica* 219, no. 3 (May–June 2005): 154–66.

22. J. R. Sparrow, et al., "Involvement of Oxidative Mechanisms in Blue-Light-Induced Damage to A2E-Laden RPE," *Investigative Ophthalmology and Visual Science* 43 (2002): 1222–27.

23. M. Boulton, et al., "Retinal Photodamage," *Journal of Photochemistry and Photobiology* B 64 (2001): 144–61.

24. M. Rozanowska, et al., "Blue Light-Induced Reactivity of Retinal Age Pigment. In Vitro Generation of Oxygen-Reactive Species," *Journal of Biological Chemistry* 270, no. 32 (August 11, 1995): 18825–30.

25. L. Verma, et al., "Phototoxic Retinopathy," *Ophthalmology Clinics of North America* 14, no. 4 (2001): 601–09.

26. A. Pawlak, et al., "Action Spectra for the Photoconsumption of Oxygen by Human Ocular Lipofuscin and Lipofuscin Extracts," *Archives of Biochemistry and Biophysics* 403, no. 1 (July 2002): 59–62.

27. E. M. Gasyna, et al., "Blue Light Induces Apoptosis in Human Fetal Retinal Pigment Epithelium," E Abstract 248 *Ophthalmology and Visual Science,* University of Chicago.

28. L. M. Rapp, and S. C. Smith, "Morphologic Comparisons between Rhodopsinmediated and Short-Wavelength Classes of Retinal Light Damage," *Investigative Ophthalmology and Visual Science* 33 (1992): 3367–77.

29. J. Mellerio, "Light Effects on the Retina," in D. M. Albert, and F. A. Jakobiec, eds., *Principles and Practice of Ophthalmology,* 1 vol. (Philadelphia: W. B. Saunders, 1994),1326–45.

30. The International Commission on Non-Ionizing Radiation Protection, "Guidelines on Limits of Exposure to Broad-Band Incoherent Optical Radiation (0.38 to 3µm)," *Health Physics* 73, no. 3 (1997): 539–54.

31. K. A. Rezaei, et al., "AcrySof Natural Filter Decreases the Blue Light Induced Apoptosis in Human Retinal Pigment Epithelium," *Ophthalmology and Visual Science,* University of Chicago.

32. G. R. Jackson, C. Owsley, E. P. Cordle, et al., "Aging and Scotopic Sensitivity," *Vision Research* 38, no. 22 (1998): 3655–62.

33. R. Mumford, "Improving Visual Efficiency with Selected Lighting," *Journal of Optometric Visual Development* 33, no. 3 (Fall 2002).

34. P. Glass, "Light and the Developing Retina," *Documenta Ophthalmologica: Advances in Ophthamology* 74, no. 3 (1990): 195–203.

35. M. Kini, et al., "Prevalence of Senile Cataract, Diabetic Retinopathy, Senile Macular Degeneration, and Open-Angle Glaucoma in the Framingham Eye Study," *American Journal of Ophthalmology* 85, no. 1 (1978): 28–34.

36. For more about the effects of lighting on the retina, see D. Roberts, "Artificial Lighting and the Blue Light Hazard," www.mdsupport.org/library/hazard.html (2004).

37. These recommendations are confirmed by the "SmartSight" patient education program of the American Academy of Ophthalmology in their educational handout at www.aao.org/patient_ed/smartsight.cfm.

38. H. R. Taylor, et al., "The Long Term Effects of Visible Light on the Eye," *Archives of Ophthalmology* 110, no. 1 (1992): 99–104.

39. I. S. Jain, P. Prasad, A. Gupta, et al., "Senile Macular Degeneration in India," *Indian Journal of Ophthalmology* 32 (1984): 343–46.

40. B. R. Hammond, B. R. Wooten, and D. M. Snodderly, "Cigarette Smoking and Retinal Carotenoids: Implications for Age-Related Macular Degeneration," *Vision Research* 36, no. 18 (September 1996): 3003–09.

41. J. R. Evans, A. E. Fletcher, and R. P. Wormald, "28,000 Cases of Age-Related Macular Degeneration Causing Visual Loss in People Aged 75 Years and Above in the United Kingdom May Be Attributable to Smoking," *British Journal of Ophthalmology* 89, no. 5 (2005): 550–53.

42. S. P. Kelly, J. Thornton, G. Lyratzopolous, et al., "Smoking and Blindness: Strong Evidence for the Link but Public Awareness Lags," *British Medical Journal* 328 (2004): 537–38.

43. J. M. Seddon, et al., "A Prospective Study of Cigarette Smoking and Age-Related Macular Degeneration in Women," *Journal of the American Medical Association* 276, no. 14 (1996): 1141–46.

44. W. G. Christen, J. E. Manson, J. M. Seddon, et al., "A Prospective Study of Cigarette Smoking and Risk of Cataract in Men," *Journal of the American Medical Association* 268, no. 8 (1992): 989–93.

45. M. E. Wright, S. T. Mayne, et al., "Development of a Comprehensive Dietary Antioxidant Index and Application to Lung Cancer Risk in a Cohort of Male Smokers," *American Journal of Epidemiology* 160, no. 1 (July 1, 2004): 68–76.

46. G. R. Chichili, et al., "Beta-Carotene Conversion into Vitamin A in Human Retinal Pigment Epithelial Cells," *Investigative Ophthalmology and Visual Science* 46, no. 10 (October 2005): 3562–69.

47. J. D. Stein, M. M. Brown, G. C. Brown, H. Hollands, and S. Sharma, "Quality of Life with Macular Degeneration: Perceptions of Patients, Clinicians, and Community Members," *British Journal of Ophthalmology* 87, no. 8 (2003): 8–12.

48. Definitions of classes (in parentheses) established by G. Rigatelli, et al., "Validation of a Clinical-Significance-Based Classification of Coronary Artery Anomalies," *Angiology* 56, no. 1 (Jan.–Feb. 2005): 25–34.

49. Stein, et al., "Qualify of Life." (See note 47.)

50. Ibid.

51. Originally published in *Contemporary Review,* 1877. Reprinted in *Lectures and Essays* (1879). Presently in print in W. K. Clifford, *The Ethics of Belief and Other Essays* (Prometheus Books, 1999).

52. Dorothy H. Stiefel, *Retinitis Pigmentosa: Dealing with the Threat of Loss* (revised version) (Corpus Christi, TX: Business of Living Publications, 1998), 36.

53. Lylas G. Mogk, MD, and Marja Mogk, PhD, *Macular Degeneration: The Complete Guide to Saving and Maximizing Your Sight* (New York: Ballantine Books, 2003), 188–94.

54. Steven M. Goldberg, OD, "Finding a Good Low Vision Specialist," MD Support, January 30, 1998, www.mdsupport.org/library/lovispec.html.

55. "Preliminary Phase III Data show Lucentis maintained or Improved Vision in Nearly 95 Percent of patients with wet age-related macular degeneration" (south San Francisco, May 23, 2005, Genentech, Inc.

56. M. Tolentino, et al., "Intravitreal Injection of VEGF Sirna Inhibits Growth and Leakage in a Non-Human Primate Laser Induced Model of CNV," *Retina: The Journal of Retinal and Vitreous Diseases* (February 18, 2004).

57. C. H. Park, and C. A. Toth, "Macular Translocation Surgery with 360-Degree Peripheral Retinectomy Following Ocular Photodynamic Therapy of Choroidal Neovascularization," *American Journal of Ophthalmology* 136, no. 5 (2003): 830–35.

58. Norman D. Radtke, MD, et al., "Vision Change after Sheet Transplant of Fetal Retina with Retinal Pigment Epithelium to a Patient with Retinitis Pigmentosa," *Archives of Ophthalmology* 122 (August 2004): 1159–65.

59. R. Joseph Olk, MD, et al., "Therapeutic Benefits of Infrared (810-Nm) Diode Laser Macular Grid Photocoagulation in Prophylactic Treatment of Nonexudative Age-Related Macular Degeneration," *Ophthalmology* 106, no. 11 (November 1999): 2082–90.

60. National Eye Institute, "Complications of AMD Prevention Trial (CAPT)," *Ophthalmology* 111 (2004): 1307–16.

61. Barbara McLaughlan, "Awareness of Age-Related Macular Degeneration and Associated Risk Factors," AMD Alliance International: Global Report 2005.

62. J. Seddon, "Latest Developments in Genetic and Nutritional Factors Associated with Age-Related Macular Degeneration," keynote speech at Vision 2005 on Tuesday, April 5, 2005.

63. S. Haines, et al., "Complement Factor H Variant Increases Risk of Age-Related Macular Degeneration," *Science* 308 (2005): 419–21.

64. A. O. Edwards, et al., "Complement Factor H Polymorphism and Age-Related Macular Degeneration," *Science* 308 (2005): 421–24.

65. G. S. Hageman, et al., "A Common Haplotype in the Complement Regulatory Gene Factor H (HF1/CFH) Predisposes Individuals to Age-Related Macular Degeneration," *Proceedings of the National Academy of Sciences* (USA) 102,no. 20 (May 2005): 7227–32.

66. R. J. Klein, et al., "Complement Factor H Polymorphism in Age-Related Macular Degeneration," *Science* 308 (2005): 385–89.

67. Jill C. Hennessey, and Janet Glover-Kerkvliet, "The Inheritance of Retinal Degenerations," booklet from the Foundation Fighting Blindness, 1995 (Owings Mills, MD), 6–7. Available for download at http://www.blindness.org/pdfs/TheInheritanceofRetinal Degenerations.pdf.

68. W. Smith, J. Assink, R. Klein, et al., "Risk Factors for Age-Related Macular Degeneration. Pooled Findings from Three Continents," *Archives of Ophthalmology* 108 (2001): 697–704.

69. M. Miyazaki, H. Nakamura, et al., "Risk Factors for Age-Related Maculopathy in a Japanese Population: The Hisayama Study," *British Journal of Ophthalmology* 87, no. 4 (2003): 469–72.

70. G. Chaine, A. Hullo, J. Sahel, et al., "Case-Control Study of the Risk Factors for Age-Related Macular Degeneration. France DMLA Study Group," *British Journal of Ophthalmology* 82, no. 9 (1998): 996–1002.

71. S. K. Law, Y. H. Sohn, D. Hoffman, et al., "Optic Disc Appearance in Advanced Age-Related Macular Degeneration," *American Journal of Ophthalmology* 138, no. 1 (July 2004): 135–36.

72. T. E. Clemons, R. C. Milton, R. Klein, J. M. Seddon, F. L. Ferris 3rd, "Age-Related Eye Disease Study Research Group," *Ophthalmology* 112, no. 4 (2005): 533–39.

73. R. N. Frank, J. E. Puklin, C. Stock, et al., "Race, Iris Color, and Age-Related Macular Degeneration," *Transactions of the American Ophthalmological Society* 98 (2000): 109–15.

74. "2004 Traffic Safety Annual Assessment—Early Results," 2004 Analysis Reporting System (FARS): August 2005. Available at www-nrd.nhtsa.dot.gov/pdf/nrd30/NCSA/RNotes/2005/809897.pdf.

75. Sara B. Vyrostek, Joseph L. Annest, PhD, and George W. Ryan, PhD, "Surveillance for Fatal and Nonfatal Injuries—United States, 2001," Centers for Disease Control 53(SS07) (September 3, 2004): Table 6. Available at http://iier.isciii.es/mmwr/preview/mmwrhtml/ss5307a1.htm.

76. Bureau of Labor Statistics, 2003. www.bts.gov/publications/national_transportation_statistics (Adjusted for gas increase to date.)

77. Ibid.

78. Joel M. Deutsch, "The Day I Quit Driving," *Los Angeles Times*, March 6, 1997, Life and Style sec.

79. For more information, see the Web site of the BiOptic Driving Network at www.biopticdriving.org.

80. C. Zell, "Friends, Neighbors and Relations: Alternative Sources for Transportation" Travel with Charlie: Lessons from Experience (Organization of Macular Friends, June 2002). Published at www.mdsupport.org/charlie/12.html.

81. "Definitions," Americans with Disabilities Act of 1990 (Pub. L. 101-336): Sec. 12102.

82. "BBB Wise Giving Alliance Standards for Charity Accountability," www.give.org/standards/newcbbbstds.asp (2003).

83. Chris I. Baker, et al., "Reorganization of Visual Processing in Macular Degeneration," *Journal of Neuroscience* 25, no. 3 (January 19, 2005): 614–18.

84. Definition of "visual," in *The American Heritage Dictionary of the English Language,* 4th edition (American Heritage, 2004).

85. Ibid, "vision"

86. *Webster's Online 1913 Dictionary* and *Princeton University's Word-Net Dictionary* (www.webster-dictionary.org).

87. D. C. Coile, "Bringing Dog Vision into Focus," *Dog World* (March 1998): 30–35.

88. Elizabeth Pennisi, "A Low Number Wins the GeneSweep Pool," *Science* 300, no. 5625 (2003): 1484.

89. Reported to the Association for Research on Ophthalmology (ARVO) annual meeting, Fort Lauderdale, Florida, year 2000, by Dr. Derek van der Kooy (University of Toronto) and Dr. Iqbal Ahmad (University of Nebraska).

90. Michael Young, MD, et al., "Multipotent Retinal Progenitors Express Developmental Markers, Differentiate into Retinal Neurons, and Preserve Light-Mediated Behavior," *Investigative Ophthalmology and Visual Science* 45 (2004):4167–73.

91. Announcement made October 2004 to the National Academy of Sciences by Derek Van der Kooy, Department of Medical Biophysics, University of Toronto, Ontario, Canada.

92. At the time of this writing, the following groups are researching artificial retinas: Optobionics Company in Chicago, the Harvard–M.I.T. Retinal Implant Project, the Intraocular Retinal Prosthesis Group at the University of Southern California, and a cooperative effort between the Stanford University School of Medicine and the Kresge Eye Institute.

93. Dr. Isaac Lipshitz and Yossi Gross, VisionCare Ophthalmic Technologies, Inc. (VisionCare), Saratoga, California and Yehud, Israel.

94. Parkinson Study Group, "What Is a Clinical Trial?" Available at www.parkinson-study-group.org.

95. By the author, as inspired by "Crossings," a poem by Lee Webber.

Acknowledgments

MY THANKS to the following people for their invaluable contributions in the way of submissions, information, advice, and review of the material contained in this book.

The AMD Internet community (members of MDList and MDForum)

Mary Jay Clough, ACSW (Jewish Guild for the Blind, New York City)

Roy G. Cole, OD, FAAO (Jewish Guild for the Blind, New York City)

K. Bailey Freund, MD (Vitreous Retina Macula Consultants of New York)

Jennifer Galbraith, OD, MS (Rebman Eye Care, Elizabethtown, Pennsylvania)

Brian Gerritsen, MA, CLVT (Low Vision Rehabilitation Services, North Ogden, Utah)

Stephen Goldberg, OD (Optometrist, St. Louis, Missouri)

Robert Hammer, B.Optom., MSc (Optometrist, Petah Tikva, Israel)

Kurt Heinmiller (SESCO Lighting, Inc., Fort Lauderdale, Florida)

Randall T. Jose, OD, FAAO (University of Houston College of Optometry)

Ron Lazarus (LazLight, Fort Lauderdale, Florida)

Joseph H. Maino, OD, FAAO (Kansas City Veterans Affairs Medical Center, Kansas City, Missouri)

Lylas G. Mogk, MD (Henry Ford Health System Visual Rehabilitation and Research Center, Grosse Pointe and Livonia, Michigan)

Martin A. Mainster, PhD, MD, FRCOphth. (University of Kansas Medical Center, Kansas City, Kansas)

Angel Pacheco (Jewish Guild for the Blind, New York City)

Seymour Rob Robins (author)

Jeff Roberts (Evayla Web Solutions, Kansas City, Missouri)

Spencer Thornton, MD (BioSyntrx, Inc., Lexington, South Carolina)

Ellen Troyer, MT, MA (BioSyntrx, Inc., Colorado Springs, Colrado)

Wendy Strouse Watt, OD (Optometrist, DuBois, Pennsylvania)

Charlie Zell (Organization of Macular Friends, Sacramento, California)

Index

Numbers preceded by an *n* (*n*37) indicates an endnote.

strobing lights, 26–27
subfoveal wet AMD, 6, 10
successful living, examples of, 78–79,
   146–49, 179–80, 204–7, 226–27
sunglasses, 28, 48, 83
Supplemental Transportation Programs
   for Seniors, 159
supplements. *See also* antioxidants; diet
   and eye health
   adverse effects from, 296
   AREDS formula, 46–47, 115
   asking doctors before taking, 113–15
   dosages, 43–44
   for retina defense systems, 49
   water-soluble versus fat-soluble, 45
   for zeaxanthin and lutein, 41–43
support. *See* family and friends; sources
   for information and help
support groups, 13–14, 73–75, 88,
   143–45
surgical treatments, 117–20
swelling of the retinal tissue, 7, 27, 33,
   34–35
symptoms of AMD, 25–29

T
TASK force
   Tenacity, 78–83
   Adaptability, 83–87
   Support, 87–88
   Knowledge, 88–89
   overview, 77–78, 89–90
tear film on cornea, 20
television magnifiers, 68
temporal (toward the ear), 36
tenacity, 78–83
TENS unit, 123–24
three Bs for better vision
   Bigger (magnification), 64–69, 86,
      228–30
   Bolder (contrast), 70–71
   Brighter (illumination), 69–70
   overview, 64, 186–87
tobacco smoke, 39, 51–52
Topamax, 290
Travatan, 295–96
traveling, 129, 176–78
Trusopt, 294–95

U
UV (ultraviolet) rays, 39, 41, 48–49, 83

V
variable expressivity of gene, 140
vascular endothelial growth factor
   (VEGF), 43, 110
verteporfin, 108
Viagra, 291
viral vectors, 216
visual, definition of, 208–9
visual field, 20, 33, 35–36, 37
visual hallucinations, 28–29
visual impairment, 3, 12–13, 59–60,
   208–9
visually-impaired person (VIP)
   congenital versus aging into, 55–57,
      211–13
   etiquette rules for friends of, 14
vision (ability to see) of, 209–13
visual symptoms of AMD, 25–29
vitamin A (beta-carotene), 45, 46,
   50–52, 296
vitamin C, 45, 46
vitamin D, 45
vitamin E, 41, 43–47, 49
vitamin K, 45
vitrectomy, 26, 119–20
vitreous fluid, 19, 21, 26

W
waves of light, 26–27
well being, research on, 53–55
wet AMD
   and AREDS formula, 47
   drug treatments for, 108–12
   and elevated homocysteine level, 45
   macular translocation for, 117–18
   overview, 3–4, 5–6, 9, 127
   preventing, 46–47
white cane, carrying a, 12–13, 127
white halogen light, 51, 69
Wilmer Eye Institute, 315*n*1
wine, 44

X
Xalatan, 295–96

Z
zeaxanthin, 41–42, 47
Zell, Charlie, 159–60
zinc, 46–47